Atlas of
Airway Management: Techniques and Tools

Steven L. Orebaugh, M.D.

Assistant Professor of Anesthesiology
Assistant Clinical Professor of Emergency Medicine
University of Pittsburgh Medical Center-Southside
Pittsburgh, Pennsylvania

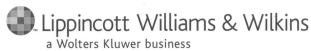
Lippincott Williams & Wilkins
a Wolters Kluwer business

Philadelphia • Baltimore • New York • London
Buenos Aires • Hong Kong • Sydney • Tokyo

Acquisitions Editor: Brian Brown
Managing Editor: Nicole Dernoski
Developmental Editor: Brigitte Wilke
Project Manager: Alicia Jackson
Senior Manufacturing Manager: Benjamin Rivera
Marketing Manager: Angela Panetta
Design Coordinator: Stephen Druding
Cover Designer: Stephen Druding
Production Service: Maryland Composition
Printer: RR Donnelly–China

Library of Congress Cataloging-in-Publication Data

Orebaugh, Steven L.
  Atlas of airway management : tools and techniques / Steven L. Orebaugh.
      p. ; cm.
  Includes bibliographical references and index.
  ISBN 978-0-7817-9724-5
  ISBN 0-7817-9724-1
  1. Airway (Medicine)—Atlases. 2. Trachea—Intubation—Atlases. 3. Artificial respiration—
Atlases. I. Title.
  [DNLM: 1. Intubation, Intratracheal—Atlases. 2. Airway Obstruction—therapy—Atlases.
3. Emergency Treatment—Atlases. 4. Laryngoscopy—Atlases.
WF 17 066a 2007]
RC732.O74 2007
616.20022′3—dc22

                                                                    2006015771

Care has been taken to confirm the accuracy of the information presented and to describe generally
accepted practices. However, the authors, editors, and publisher are not responsible for errors or
omissions or for any consequences from application of the information in this book and make no
warranty, expressed or implied, with respect to the currency, completeness, or accuracy of the
contents of the publication. Application of the information in a particular situation remains the
professional responsibility of the practitioner.

The authors, editors, and publisher have exerted every effort to ensure that drug selection and dosage
set forth in this text are in accordance with current recommendations and practice at the time of
publication. However, in view of ongoing research, changes in government regulations, and the con-
stant flow of information relating to drug therapy and drug reactions, the reader is urged to check the
package insert for each drug for any change in indications and dosage and for added warnings and
precautions. This is particularly important when the recommended agent is a new or infrequently
employed drug.

Some drugs and medical devices presented in the publication have Food and Drug Administration
(FDA) clearance for limited use in restricted research settings. It is the responsibility of the health
care provider to ascertain the FDA status of each drug or device planned for use in their clinical
practice.

To purchase additional copies of this book, call our customer service department at (800) 638-3030
or fax orders to (301) 223-2320. International customers should call (301) 223-2300.

Visit Lippincott Williams & Wilkins on the Internet: at LWW.com. Lippincott Williams & Wilkins
customer service representatives are available from 8:30 am to 6 pm, EST.

8 7 6 5 4 3

Dedication

Dedicated to my wife, Jennifer, and my daughter, Olivia.

Acknowledgments

I greatly acknowledge the help of Dr. Branton Barstetter, of the University of Pittsburgh Medical Center Department of Radiology, for providing the radiologic images in Chapter 11; Alison Yeung, DDS, and Dr. William Chung of the Oromaxillofacial Surgery Division of UPMC for photos of oral pathology in Chapter 11; and Samuel Tisherman, MD, of the Department of Surgery at UPMC for photos of surgical airway in Chapter 33. Also, I wish to thank Stephen Schiller and Karl Storz, Endoscopy, Inc., for generously providing video and digital imaging equipment, fiberoptic brochoscopes, and video laryngoscopes. Thanks also for LMA of North America, Mercury Medical, King Medical, Tyco Healthcare, Engineered Medical Systems, and Achi medical products for providing high quality images of their products. I must recognize the anesthesiologists and nurse anesthetists of the University of Pittsburgh Medical Center-Southside who enthusiastically assisted in preparation of photographs for this book, the anesthesiology residents and medical students from the University of Pittsburgh who likewise facilitated the process of obtaining clinical photographs and photos of simulated airway management scenarios, and John McCaulley, medical photographer, who provided much of his time and effort to help bring this idea to fruition.

Preface

My aim in creating this book is to assist those learning to manage the airway to understand the basics—mask ventilation and optimal direct laryngoscopy—as well as to comprehend alternative techniques for situations in which direct laryngoscopy is difficult, or cannot be utilized. There is an ever-expanding array of airway tools, of many different types, covering a spectrum of costs and degrees of complexity. It behooves the provider to understand how different techniques work and when they are effective so that two or three alternatives to laryngoscopy can be chosen, learned, and practiced. Because I initially trained in emergency medicine, then critical care medicine and, finally, anesthesiology, I have experienced airway management from several different viewpoints. I have attempted to share these perspectives in this atlas.

Many fine airway management books exist, ranging from small handbooks to expansive texts. Some of these texts suffer from a lack of instructive illustration. In an attempt to complement them, this atlas was created, and thus provides more illustration than text. In order to make the relationships between anatomy and airway management tools clear, a large variety of illustrations is presented, including mockups in cadaver specimens, photos of airway management in the clinical setting, simulated airway management scenarios, and photographs of the airway utilizing video laryngoscopes and fiberoptic bronchoscopes.

Most of the atlas is dedicated to defining and illustrating the many devices and techniques that exist for endotracheal intubation when direct laryngoscopy is difficult or undesirable. These topics are covered in eight parts, in the following areas: adjuncts to direct laryngoscopy, blind intubation techniques, light-guided intubation, retrograde intubation, fiberoptic techniques, emergency ventilation techniques (supraglottic and infraglottic), combinations of techniques, and emergency surgical airways. Within each section are one to five chapters detailing the devices or procedures that fall under that heading.

The first portion of this atlas is intended to cover basic airway management, including airway anatomy, bag-mask ventilation, direct laryngoscopy, and pharmacology relevant to endotracheal intubation. While the purpose of this book is to provide information on management of the adult airway, a chapter on the pediatric airway is included. When applicable, references to pediatric airway management are made in the various chapters covering implements or techniques. In the second section, difficult airway management is explored, including the epidemiology of this life-threatening problem in elective cases in operating room, and in more emergent settings. Decision-making in the face of recognized or potential difficult airways, due to anatomy, disease, or obesity, for example, is discussed, as well as training of physicians, students, and nurses at the University of Pittsburgh utilizing high fidelity human simulation. In the last chapter of this section, a survey of anatomic and pathologic causes of difficult airway management is presented.

Brevity and an organized format for the text are as important in an atlas as are the illustrations themselves. For this reason, the chapters covering specific tools or techniques are arranged according to the following template: The concept is presented, followed by a discussion of existing evidence supporting the use of the intervention. Next, the preparatory steps for the procedure are listed, followed by a description of the steps necessary to carry out the procedure itself. Following this is a listing of elements of practicality, affordability, portability, familiarity, complexity, and other concerns which impact the ability to integrate the tool or technique into medical practice. Finally, indications, contraindications, and complications of the intervention are noted. A series of illustrations is provided, showing the tool(s) involved, how these are placed in the patient (demonstrated in a cadaver specimen), and clinical photos, or simulations, of the device in use. When appropriate, step-by-step sequential illustrations show the progression of the procedure.

Steven L. Orebaugh, MD
Assistant Professor of Anesthesiology
Assistant Clinical Professor of Emergency Medicine
University of Pittsburgh Medical Center, Southside

Table of Contents

Airway Anatomy

In managing the airway, knowledge of anatomic structures and their relationships can assist the laryngoscopist in a number of ways. It is important to apply this understanding in overcoming airway obstruction during loss of consciousness, in providing adequate exposure of the glottis during direct laryngoscopy, and in the application of various tools and adjuncts when direct laryngoscopy proves difficult or impossible. Externally, important landmarks include the hyoid bone, cephalad to the larynx, and the large, unpaired cartilages of the larynx. These consist of the shield-shaped thyroid cartilage (or "Adam's apple") and the signet ring-shaped cricoid cartilage below it. Between these cartilages lies the cricothyroid interval, through which several emergency airway devices can be placed. Below the cricoid cartilage, the tracheal rings are palpable (Fig. 1.1).

During direct laryngoscopy, while viewing the glottis from above, several features are apparent (Fig. 1.2). The vestibular folds, or false cords, lie above the true vocal folds. The vocal folds, or true cords, may or may not be well-visualized when the glottic opening is exposed. The laryngeal introitus is bounded anteriorly by the epiglottis, laterally by the aryepiglottic folds on both sides, and posteriorly by the protuberances of the paired corniculate and arytenoid cartilages, with the arytenoid notch in the midline between them.

In a sagittal and a coronal cross-section of the larynx (Figs. 1.3 and 1.4), it can be seen that the vocal ligaments traverse the distance between the thyroid cartilage, anteriorly, and the arytenoid cartilages, which are perched atop the cricoid cartilage, posteriorly. The arytenoids serve as a point of origin for several intrinsic laryngeal muscles, which move the true vocal cords to produce phonation. Inferior to the vocal folds is the circumferential ring of the cricoid cartilage. Its inferior aspect marks the proximal tracheal lumen.

In the supine position, during unconsciousness, relaxation of the muscles supporting the airway frequently leads to upper airway obstruction (Fig. 1.5). This occurs primarily at the level of the soft palate and tongue, and can usually be overcome by jaw thrust, chin lift, "sniffing" position, or insertion of an oropharyngeal or nasopharyngeal airway.

A number of structures may obstruct the laryngoscopist's view of the laryngeal inlet. Figure 1.6, a cadaver specimen sectioned in the sagittal plane, makes apparent the difficulty. Mouth opening at the temporomandibular joint, oral cavity size, dental structures, and tongue size are immediately apparent as obstructions to visualization of the glottis. Furthermore, the angle at which one attempts to bring the airway entrance into view is of importance. In neutral position, the line of sight reaches the posterior pharynx, uvula, and soft palate. With extension, it is possible to view the hypopharynx, the area just cephalad to the glottic opening. When the patient's head is placed in the sniffing position (flexion of the cervical spine and extension of the atlanto-occipital joint), the axes of the airway are better aligned. This has become the standard patient position for optimizing the view of the airway during direct laryngoscopy (see Chapter 3).

Innervation of the key airway structures is depicted in Figure 1.7. The internal branch of the superior laryngeal nerve innervates the laryngeal mucosa above the vocal folds, including that of the laryngeal surface of the epiglottis. Above this level, the glossopharyngeal nerve is responsible for sensation in the posterior tongue, vallecula, and pharynx, while the lingual nerve, a branch of Cranial Nerve VII, supplies sensation to the anterior tongue. The afferent limb of the gag reflex is primarily served by the glossopharyngeal nerve, and the muscles of the pharynx, innervated by the vagus nerve, enact the efferent limb. Below the level of the vocal cords, the recurrent laryngeal nerves supply sensation. All of the intrinsic muscles of the larynx are innervated by the recurrent laryngeal nerve, with the exception of the cricothyroid muscles, which are innervated by the external branch of the superior laryngeal nerve. Understanding these innervation patterns is useful when providing topical anesthesia or nerve blocks for awake intubation utilizing a fiberoptic bronchoscope.

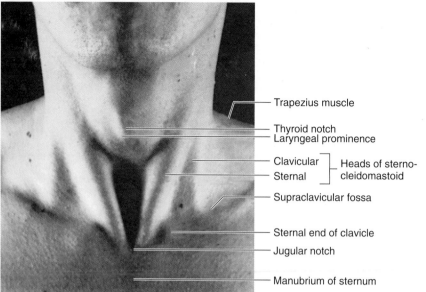

Figure 1.1 Surface anatomy of the larynx and surrounding structures.

Trapezius muscle

Thyroid notch
Laryngeal prominence

Clavicular
Sternal ─ Heads of sterno-cleidomastoid

Supraclavicular fossa

Sternal end of clavicle

Jugular notch

Manubrium of sternum

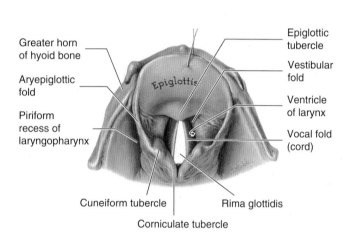

Greater horn
of hyoid bone

Aryepiglottic
fold

Piriform
recess of
laryngopharynx

Epiglottis

Epiglottic
tubercle

Vestibular
fold

Ventricle
of larynx

Vocal fold
(cord)

Cuneiform tubercle

Rima glottidis

Corniculate tubercle

Figure 1.2 Superior view of the laryngeal introitus.

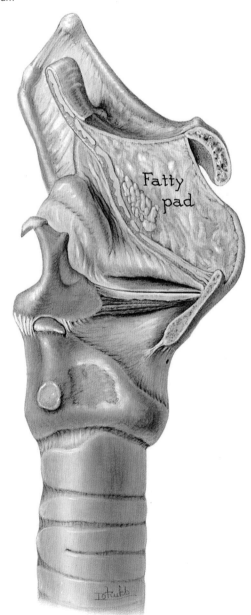

Fatty
pad

Figure 1.3 Sagittal section through the larynx.

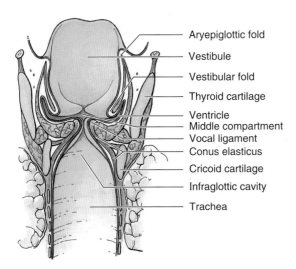

Figure 1.4 Coronal section through the larynx.

- Aryepiglottic fold
- Vestibule
- Vestibular fold
- Thyroid cartilage
- Ventricle
- Middle compartment
- Vocal ligament
- Conus elasticus
- Cricoid cartilage
- Infraglottic cavity
- Trachea

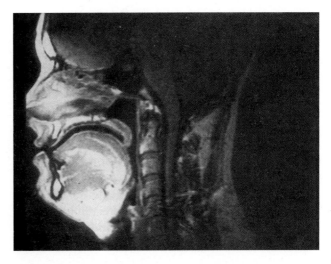

Figure 1.5 MRI of unconscious (sedated) patient, showing airway obstruction at level of soft palate. (From Mathru M, Esch O, Lang J, et al. Magnetic resonance imaging of the upper airway. *Anesthesiology* 1996;84:273–279, with permission.)

Figure 1.6 **A.** Sagittal section through cadaver head, showing anatomy of airway and surrounding structures.

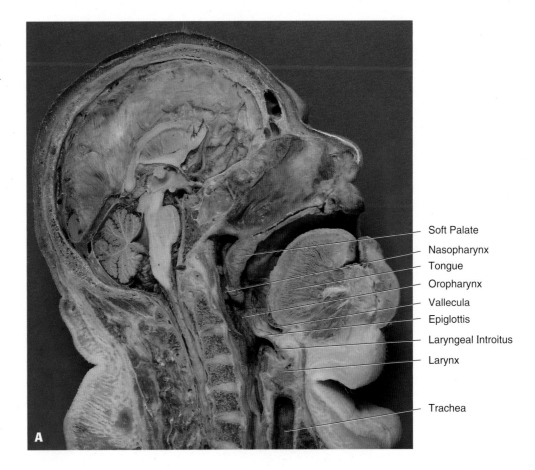

- Soft Palate
- Nasopharynx
- Tongue
- Oropharynx
- Vallecula
- Epiglottis
- Laryngeal Introitus
- Larynx
- Trachea

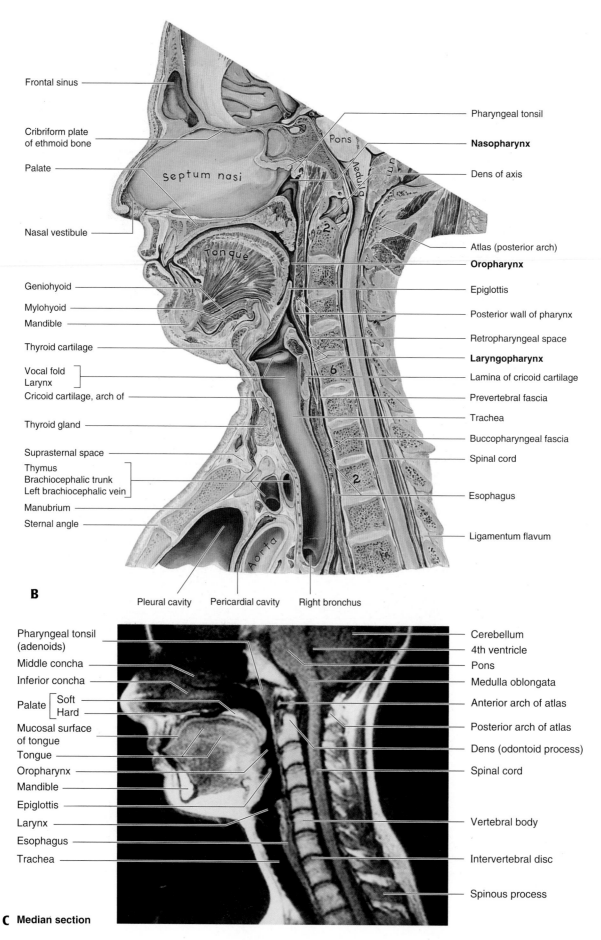

Frontal sinus

Cribriform plate
of ethmoid bone

Palate

Septum nasi

Nasal vestibule

Tongue

Geniohyoid

Mylohyoid

Mandible

Thyroid cartilage

Vocal fold
Larynx

Cricoid cartilage, arch of

Thyroid gland

Suprasternal space

Thymus
Brachiocephalic trunk
Left brachiocephalic vein

Manubrium

Sternal angle

Pons

Medulla

Aorta

Pharyngeal tonsil

Nasopharynx

Dens of axis

Atlas (posterior arch)

Oropharynx

Epiglottis

Posterior wall of pharynx

Retropharyngeal space

Laryngopharynx

Lamina of cricoid cartilage

Prevertebral fascia

Trachea

Buccopharyngeal fascia

Spinal cord

Esophagus

Ligamentum flavum

B

Pleural cavity   Pericardial cavity   Right bronchus

Pharyngeal tonsil
(adenoids)

Middle concha

Inferior concha

Palate Soft
        Hard

Mucosal surface
of tongue

Tongue

Oropharynx

Mandible

Epiglottis

Larynx

Esophagus

Trachea

Cerebellum

4th ventricle

Pons

Medulla oblongata

Anterior arch of atlas

Posterior arch of atlas

Dens (odontoid process)

Spinal cord

Vertebral body

Intervertebral disc

Spinous process

C Median section

Figure 1.6 (*continued*) **B.** Sagittal section of head-neck showing laryngeal and pharyngeal structures. **C.** Sagittal MRI of head/neck showing laryngeal and pharyngeal structures.

Figure 1.7 Innervation of the larynx. (From Moore KL, Dalley AF. *Clinically oriented anatomy*, 4th ed. Philadelphia: Lippincott Williams & Wilkins; 1999, with permission.)

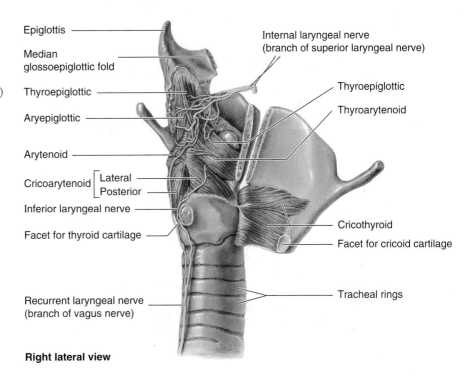

Epiglottis

Median glossoepiglottic fold

Thyroepiglottic

Aryepiglottic

Arytenoid

Cricoarytenoid [Lateral / Posterior]

Inferior laryngeal nerve

Facet for thyroid cartilage

Recurrent laryngeal nerve (branch of vagus nerve)

Internal laryngeal nerve (branch of superior laryngeal nerve)

Thyroepiglottic

Thyroarytenoid

Cricothyroid

Facet for cricoid cartilage

Tracheal rings

Right lateral view

REFERENCES:

1. Adnet F, Borran SW, Dumas JL, et al. Study of "sniffing position" by magnetic resonance imaging. *Anesthesiology* 2001; 24:83–86.
2. Mathru M, Esch O, Lang J, et al. Magnetic resonance imaging of the upper airway. *Anesthesiology* 1996;84:273–279.
3. Evans R, Crawford MW, Noseworthy M, et al. Effect of increasing depth of propofol anesthesia on upper airway configuration in children. *Anesthesiology* 2003;99:596–602.
4. Isomo S. Common practice and concepts in anesthesia: time for reassessment. *Anesthesiology* 2001;95:825–827.
5. Moore KL, Dalley AF. *Clinical anatomy*, 4th ed. Philadelphia: Lippincott Williams & Wilkins; 1999:995–1081.

2

Mask Ventilation

Concept: Mask ventilation is an effective, noninvasive means of providing ventilation and oxygenation in the decompensated or unconscious patient. Maintenance of a patent airway with mask ventilation is an important skill that requires understanding and experience to perform well. Furthermore, the ability to ventilate by mask is life-supporting or even life-saving when direct laryngoscopy proves difficult. In some scenarios, ventilation by mask may be all the airway management necessary to ensure temporary oxygenation and ventilation, while a reversible condition is addressed, and the patient is expected to then resume spontaneous ventilation. When endotracheal intubation is necessary in the elective, fasted setting, as in the operating room, initial ventilation with the face mask should precede attempts at intubation in the apneic patient. However, in emergent airway management scenarios, face mask ventilation is withheld to avert gastric insufflation and the potential for regurgitation ("rapid sequence induction" or "rapid sequence intubation"). An assortment of face masks for ventilation is shown in Figure 2.1. Clear masks are preferred to other types, so that regurgitation or vomitus is immediately apparent.

Evidence: Effective mask ventilation requires an open airway and a tight seal between the mask and the face. Patency of the airway can be optimized with a "triple airway maneuver" in which chin lift, head extension, and mouth opening are provided. Placement of the patient in "sniffing position," with the cervical spine flexed and the head extended, also contributes to this. Mask fit can be optimized with the choice of mask shape, and with appropriate inflation of the air-filled bladder, or cushion, which surrounds most modern ventilation masks. As the mask is placed over the mouth and nose, it is imperative that pressure is applied from above as the jaw is lifted into the mask. This is most effectively performed by utilizing the thumb and forefinger of the left hand to apply the mask, while the remaining fingers pull the boney mandible upward. This chin lift-jaw thrust maneuver prevents the soft tissue obstruction of the airway that will occur if the mandible is displaced in a posterior direction with mask pressure in the unconscious patient, or if the fingers apply pressure to the floor of the mouth, obstructing the oral cavity (1). It is particularly useful to "hook" the fifth finger behind the angle of the mandible to aid in lifting it upward.

Mask ventilation also necessitates a source of pressure to move gas into the airway. Depending upon the setting, the oxygen source in bag-mask ventilation may be a hospital wall source, oxygen tank with regulator, or an anesthesia machine and circuit. Effective ventilation is confirmed by visible chest rise and audible breath sounds, as well as the presence of exhaled CO_2, if monitored (as is typical in the operating room). High inflation pressures (more than 20 cm to 25 cm H_2O) may contribute to gastric insufflation and regurgitation, and should be avoided if possible. If such high pressures are required, obstruction of the airway should be suspected, although poor lung and/or chest wall compliance are also possible causes.

Airway obstruction in the unconscious individual is usually attributed to relaxation of the tongue, with posterior displacement of its muscular mass, occluding the airway at oropharyngeal levels. Studies with magnetic resonance imaging in sedated adults suggest that the soft palate plays a very important, and perhaps predominant, role in this phenomenon (2). Doubtless, both mechanisms may contribute, and overcoming this obstruction is paramount in ensuring oxygenation and ventilation. Either oropharyngeal or nasopharyngeal airways should be utilized to complement mask ventilation when obstruction occurs, and if ineffective, may be used together (Figs. 2.2 to 2.7). Both of these aids must be sized appropriately, or they may be ineffective, or even make obstruction worse.

At times, mask ventilation may remain difficult or impossible despite optimal technique (Figs. 2.8 and 2.9), even with the use of nasal and/or oral airways. Difficult mask ventilation may occur in up to 5% of cases, but impossible mask ventilation is much less common (3,4). Under these circumstances, assistance should be obtained and a two-handed, two-person mask technique with jaw thrust should be utilized in an attempt to provide some degree of ventilation (Fig. 2.10). If only unskilled assistance is available (i.e., no experience in airway management), then the provider in charge of the airway should use both hands to secure the mask seal, while his/her assistant squeezes the anesthesia bag or resuscitation bag (Fig. 2.11).

Figure 2.1 Examples of face masks for bag-mask ventilation.

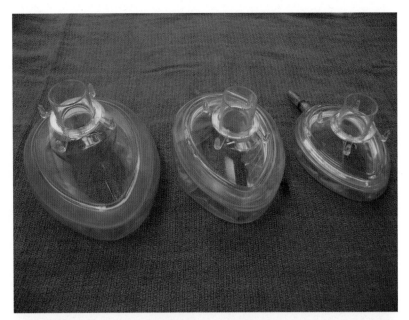

Figure 2.2 An array of oropharyngeal airways to assist with bag-mask ventilation.

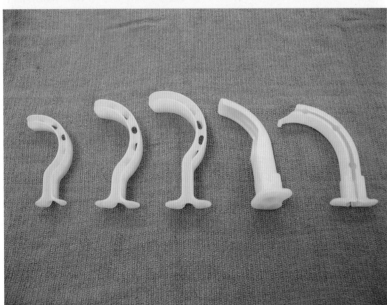

Figure 2.3 An array of nasopharyngeal airways to assist with bag-mask ventilation.

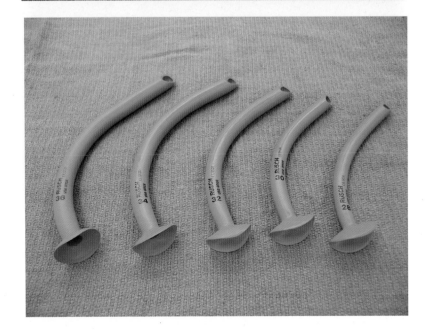

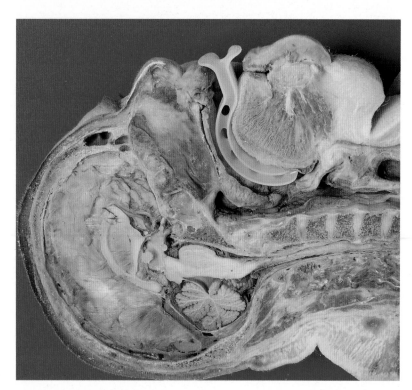

Figure 2.4 Proper placement of an oropharyngeal airway, showing effective separation of dorsal tongue from posterior oropharyngeal wall.

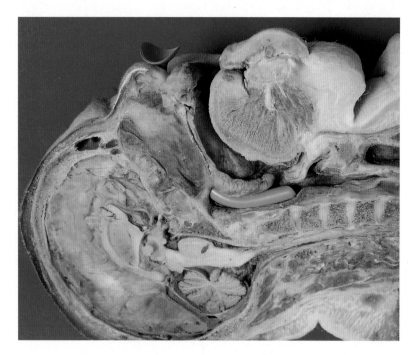

Figure 2.5 Proper placement of a nasopharyngeal airway, showing effective separation of soft palate from posterior wall of nasopharynx.

Figure 2.6 Improper size and placement of oropharyngeal airway, showing potential increase in obstruction from tongue displacement.

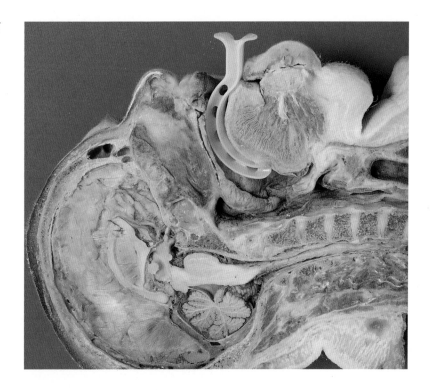

Figure 2.7 Improper size of nasopharyngeal airway, showing failed separation of soft palate from nasopharyngeal wall.

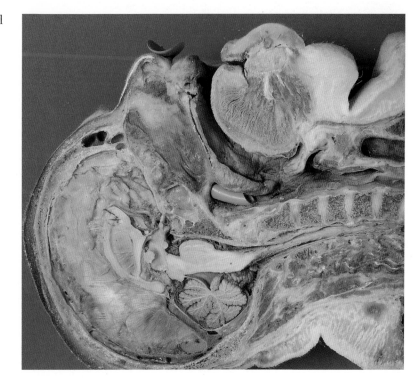

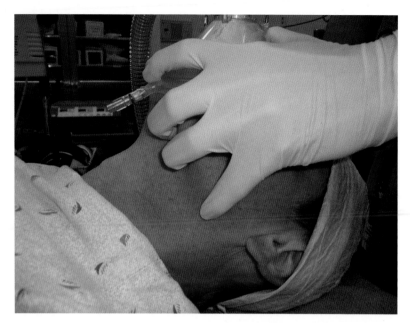

Figure 2.8 Effective application of the face mask in the unconscious patient, with thumb and forefinger holding mask to face, while the other three fingers pull the mandible up into the mask, creating seal and enacting a chin lift-jaw thrust maneuver simultaneously.

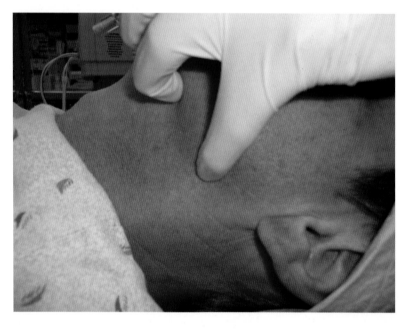

Figure 2.9 Detail of application of face mask, showing fifth finger "hooked" behind the mandibular angle, pulling mandible upward into mask.

Figure 2.10 Effective two-person mask technique allows the most skilled provider to perform a two-handed mask seal with jaw thrust, while the second operator uses one hand to enhance mask seal and the second to squeeze the bag. This technique should be employed with oral and/or nasal airways in place to optimize ventilation attempts.

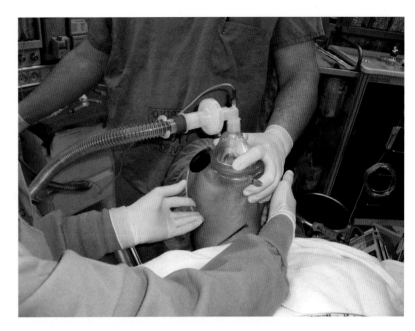

Figure 2.11 When only one skilled provider is available, he/she should place both hands on the mask, providing an effective seal, while the unskilled assistant squeezes the bag.

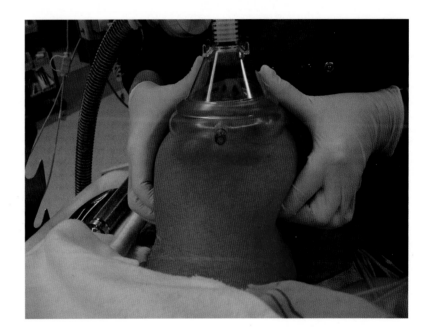

Preparation:

  Attach bag-mask apparatus to oxygen source
  Assure flow of oxygen
  Select face mask of correct size and attach to bag-mask
    or anesthesia circuit
  Place patient in optimal position: neck flexion, head
    extension ("sniffing" position)

Procedure (Figs. 2.2 to 2.11):

  Open the airway with "triple airway maneuver:" head
    extension, mouth opening, chin lift (in some
    patients, this may be all that is required to resume
    ventilation)

Place mask on face, utilizing thumb and forefinger of
  left hand on mask, and remaining three fingers on
  boney mandible, elevating it into the mask
Squeeze the bag with the right hand, until chest rise is
  evident
Ensure optimal seal of the mask on the face: leakage of
  gas should not occur with inflation pressures up to
  25 cm H_2O
If seal is inadequate, reposition mask, or change to a
  different size mask
If seal is intact, but ventilation is ineffective, suspect
  airway obstruction and place oropharyngeal or
  nasopharyngeal airway

Confirm adequate ventilation with chest rise, humidification in mask, symmetric breath sounds on auscultation, and presence of expired CO_2 (if capnometry is available)

Practicality: Simple, inexpensive, portable airway support maneuver

Requires considerable practice and experience to perform well

Indications: Altered mental status with inadequate or obstructed ventilation

Unconscious patient with apnea or inadequate ventilation

Cardiac arrest

Pre-oxygenation before intubation attempts

Ventilation after induction of anesthesia in elective surgical cases, preceding placement of endotracheal tube or laryngeal mask airway

Administration of anesthesia gases throughout certain surgical cases

Contraindications: Full stomach or risk for regurgitation (however, if hypoxemia occurs, the theoretical risk of aspiration is outweighed by the real occurrence of tissue injury from hypoxia: mask ventilation should be carried out with cricoid pressure)

Potential cervical spine injury (avoid cervical flexion or head extension: manual, in-line immobilization should be applied before attempts at direct laryngoscopy)

Severe facial trauma, precluding mask placement or seal

Upper airway foreign body obstruction: attempts should be made to clear the airway first with appropriate abdominal or chest thrusts

Complications: Ineffective ventilation with hypoxia and/or hypercarbia

Gastric insufflation

Regurgitation/aspiration of gastric contents

Trauma or bleeding from oral or nasal airways

Laryngospasm, bronchospasm or vomiting due to stimulation from oral or nasal airways (especially if placed too deeply)

REFERENCES:

1. McGee JP, Vender JS. Nonintubation management of the airway: mask ventilation. In: Benumof JL, ed. *Airway management: principles and practice.* St. Louis: Mosby; 1996: 228–254.
2. Mathru M, Esch O, Lang J, et al. Magnetic resonance imaging of the upper airway. *Anesthesiology* 1996;84:273–279.
3. Han R, Tremper KK, Kheterpal S, et al. Grading scale for mask ventilation. *Anesthesiology* 2004;101:267.
4. Langeron O, Masso E, Huraux C, et al. Prediction of difficult mask ventilation. *Anesthesiology* 2000;92:1229–1236.

Direct Laryngoscopy

Concept: When face mask ventilation is inadequate to provide necessary airway support, or when long term positive pressure ventilation is required, an endotracheal tube (ETT) should be placed. In most circumstances, direct laryngoscopy is the simplest and most readily applied means of placing the ETT. Indications for direct laryngoscopy and endotracheal intubation are summarized below.

During direct laryngoscopy the provider must bring his/her line of sight into alignment with the glottic opening in order to facilitate visualization of ETT placement. Most sources recommend that the oral, pharyngeal, and laryngeal axes be aligned by the process of patient positioning and direct laryngoscopy, to guarantee the best view of the glottic opening. However, even if one cannot peer down the laryngeal axis into the trachea, placement of the endotracheal tube is usually readily accomplished if the laryngeal inlet is visible. Evaluation of the alignment of the oral, pharyngeal, and laryngeal axes utilizing magnetic resonance imaging when the head and neck are in neutral position, in simple extension, or in "sniffing position," reveals that these three lines seldom, if ever, become well-aligned (Fig. 3.1) (1).

The forces brought to bear on the soft tissues of the oral cavity and pharynx in direct laryngoscopy must be appropriately directed. Whether a curved or straight laryngoscope blade is utilized, the operator should lift upward and away from himself/herself, a stressful maneuver that requires practice, and when prolonged, causes fatigue. When the laryngoscopist pulls towards himself/herself to create mechanical advantage, he/she is creating leverage, but the upper teeth are often contacted and in danger of injury. This maneuver is common among trainees learning laryngoscopy and must be actively discouraged.

Evidence: An important objective in direct laryngoscopy is to displace superiorly those structures that impede the view of the airway on its anterior aspect, including the tongue, floor of the mouth, mandible, and epiglottis, while positioning the head optimally so that structures posterior to the line of site are not obstacles to visualizing the larynx (2). While investigation to establish the ideal position for laryngoscopy is ongoing, it remains a standard to place the patient to undergo laryngoscopy in the sniffing position,

unless the potential of cervical spine trauma prevents this. Suboptimal views are not rare, and changes in head position may be helpful to improve visualization. Some investigators have described improved laryngoscopic views when additional cervical flexion, beyond the standard sniffing position, is utilized (3). Schmitt et al evaluated the impact of cervical flexion (beyond the usual sniffing position) in 21 patients who presented a grade 3 view at direct laryngoscopy after induction of anesthesia (4). This additional flexion was provided by an assistant who also imposed external laryngeal pressure while lifting the head and flexing the neck. The authors reported that the laryngoscopic view improved to grade 2 in more than 90% of patients with use of this maneuver.

Perhaps the best means of coping with suboptimal laryngoscopic views is to prevent their occurrence altogether. This requires that the initial attempt at direct laryngoscopy be optimal, in order to avoid repeated attempts at intubation. More than three or four failed placements of the ETT in the pharynx or laryngeal introitus may cause bleeding and supraglottic swelling, leading to a vicious cycle in which each attempt leads to a greater likelihood of failed intubation and, eventually, ventilation (5). Optimizing laryngoscopy requires that the patient is positioned appropriately for the best laryngeal view; that effective muscle relaxation is carried out with an appropriate dose of neuromuscular blocking agents (see Chapter 7); that an appropriate retraction blade is utilized to fit the situation; and that external laryngeal pressure is utilized whenever the view of the larynx is poor (5).

Most physicians prefer to initiate direct laryngoscopy with a curved blade. However, certain situations, such as prominent "buck" incisors, over-riding maxillary teeth, or a floppy epiglottis, may benefit from substitution of the straight blade. In addition, when a poor laryngeal view is evident with use of the curved blade, switching to the "paraglossal straight blade" technique may allow a substantially improved view of the glottis (6). Henderson described the use of this technique, in which the straight blade is introduced along the lateral aspect of the tongue, in 10 cases of unexpected difficult intubation with the MacIntosh blade. He reported an improved visualization of the glottis and successful intubation of the trachea in all cases.

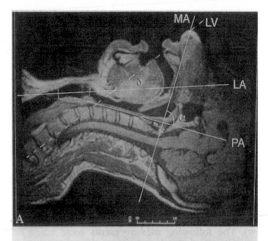

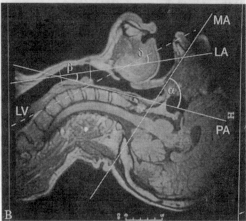

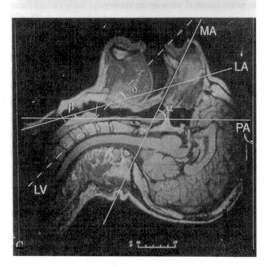

Figure 3.1 These MRI images show the alignment of the oral, pharyngeal, and laryngeal axes in neutral position, in simple head extension, and in sniffing position. (From Adnet F. Study of the "sniffing position" by magnetic resonance imaging. *Anesthesiology* 2001;94:83–86, with permission.)

In the application of external laryngeal pressure (ELP), the right hand of the laryngoscopist is placed upon the thyroid cartilage during suspension of the mandible with the retraction blade, before the endotracheal tube is held with this hand. Pressure is exerted upon the thyroid (not cricoid) cartilage with the thumb and index finger, to bring the larynx posteriorly (toward the cervical spine) and into view, nullifying the upward force that laryngoscopy may have had on the glottic structures. The glottis may also be manipulated superiorly, or from side-to-side, to improve the view (7). Once the view has been optimized, an assistant places his or her thumb and finger in exactly the same position, maintaining the relationship of anatomic structures, while the laryngoscopist grasps the ETT with his or her right hand and places it through the glottic opening. This maneuver is rapidly learned, and has been shown to substantially improve the laryngoscopic view in most patients (8).

The first attempt at direct laryngoscopy is likely to be the best attempt when these four factors are taken into account: positioning, muscle relaxation, the correct blade, and external pressure on the larynx. Precious seconds then will not be lost to correct suboptimal aspects of the procedure after a poor view of the laryngeal orifice becomes evident.

Preparation for Direct Laryngoscopy (Figs. 3.2 and 3.3):

Obtain reliable intravenous access

Appropriate pharmacological agents for induction of anesthesia and muscle relaxation (see Chapter 7) must be available

Assure suction apparatus is present and functional

Array appropriate tools for laryngoscopy, including laryngoscope with desired blade, ETT of desired size with lubricated malleable stylet, in hockey-stick configuration

Ensure proper function of laryngoscope light, and cuff of endotracheal tube

Test oxygen source, and bag-mask apparatus (either Ambu resuscitation bag or anesthesia circuit and bag)

Ensure appropriate patient monitoring is initiated (electrocardiograph, noninvasive blood pressure and pulse oximetry monitors)

Place patient in sniffing position, unless contraindications exist

Assure a means for ongoing ventilation, if long-term ventilation is expected

Have available a means to detect expiratory CO_2, for ensuring proper endotracheal tube placement in the airway

Procedure for Direct Laryngoscopy (Figs. 3.4 to 3.15):

Pre-oxygenate the patient before he/she is rendered unconscious, if possible

Figure 3.2 Appropriate "sniffing" position for direct laryngoscopy.

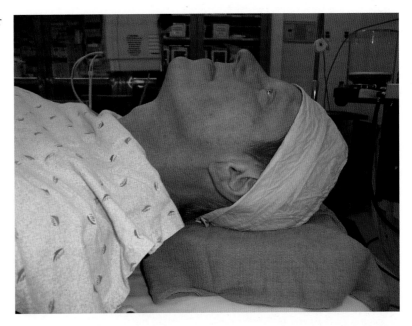

Figure 3.3 Intubation equipment.

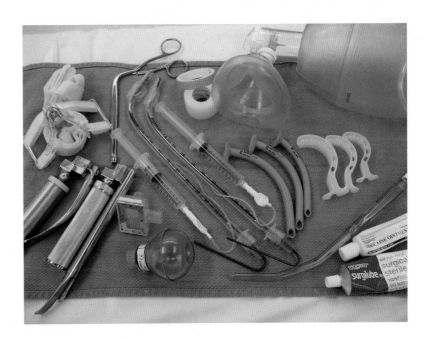

Administer hypnotic agent (unless awake intubation is planned, or patient is unconscious)

Ventilate by bag-mask after patient is apneic (unless risk of aspiration is present)

Administer muscle relaxant

Allow time for relaxant to affect airway muscles

Open mouth, using fingers or head extension

Sweep tongue to left with blade, whether straight or curved

Place the laryngoscopic blade in its appropriate position (see Chapter 4) and lift up and away to expose glottis

Utilize external laryngeal pressure, if needed, to improve view

Place the endotracheal tube in the glottic opening

Have assistant remove stylet (if used), while practitioner holds tube firmly in place

Advance the ETT another 3 cm to 4 cm

Inflate the cuff of the tube

Attach resuscitation bag or anesthesia circuit and begin ventilation

Confirm the position of the ETT with CO_2 detection, auscultation of symmetric breath sounds, and visual evidence of chest rise

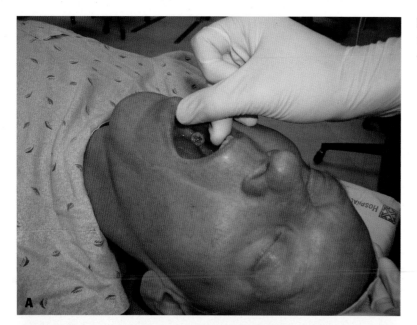

Figure 3.4 **A.** Mouth opening using fingers in a "scissors" configuration. **B.** Mouth opening using head extension.

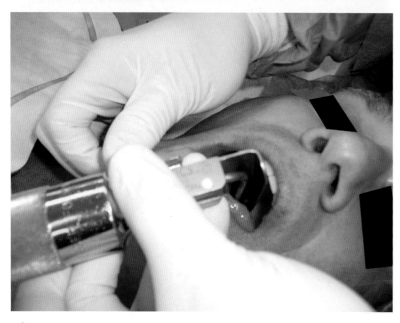

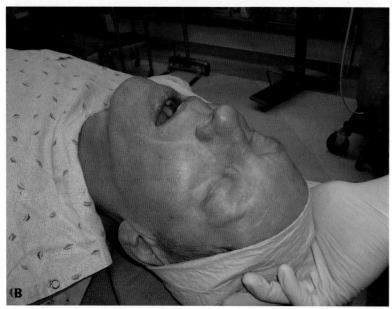

Figure 3.5 Sweeping tongue to left with laryngoscope blade.

Figure 3.6 Obstacles to visualizing the glottis: tongue, epiglottis.

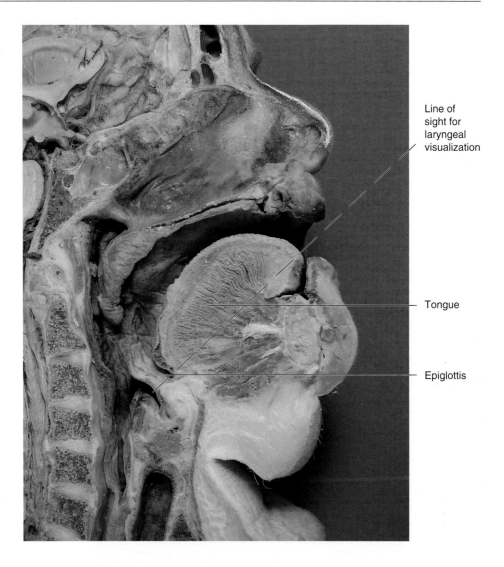

Line of sight for laryngeal visualization

Tongue

Epiglottis

Figure 3.7 Direction of forces applied for direct laryngoscopy.

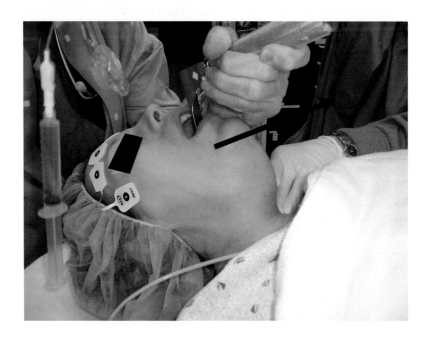

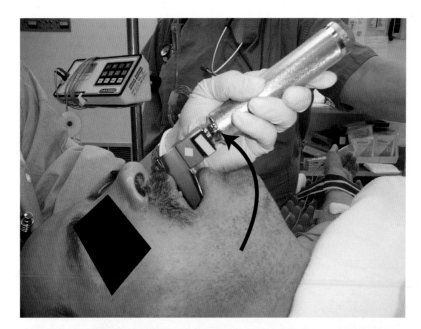

Figure 3.8 Inappropriate "levering" force in direct laryngoscopy. Note pressure of flange of MacIntosh blade against upper lip and teeth.

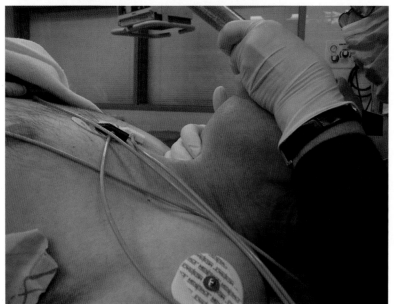

Figure 3.9 External laryngeal pressure.

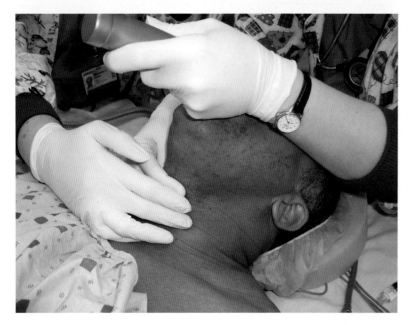

Figure 3.10 External laryngeal pressure by assistant.

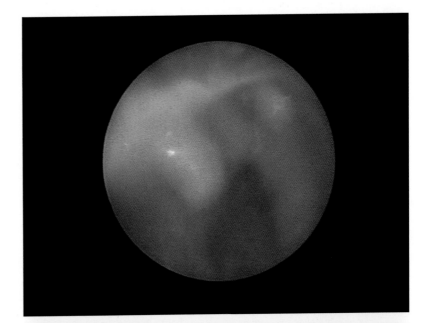

Figure 3.11 View of glottis without external laryngeal pressure.

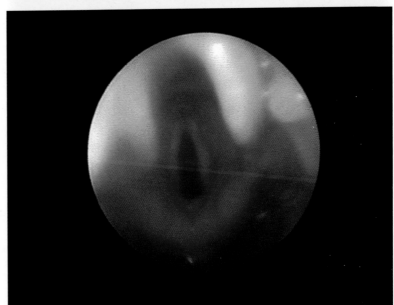

Figure 3.12 View of glottis with external laryngeal pressure.

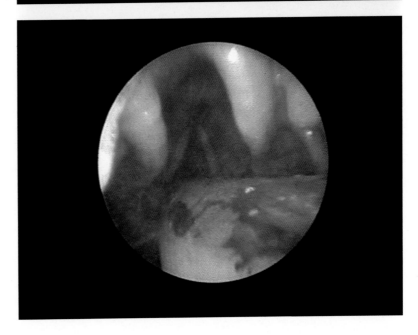

Figure 3.13 Endotracheal tube insertion.

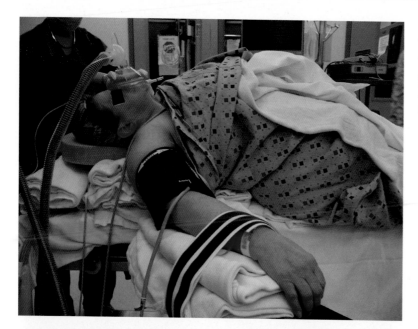

Figure 3.14 For obese patients, a "ramp" of blankets, or commercially available foam wedge, allows the patient to more effectively adopt a "sniffing" position, enabling laryngoscope blade insertion and effective direct laryngoscopy.

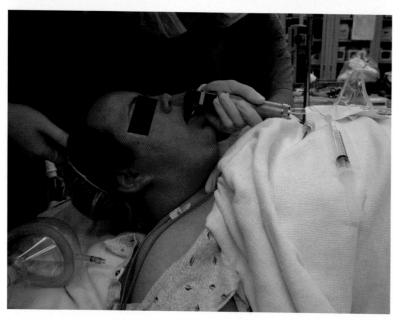

Figure 3.15 When the view during direct laryngoscopy is poor, it may be improved with the aid of an assistant, who lifts the head with the right hand, increasing the degree of cervical spine flexion, while applying external laryngeal pressure with the left hand, as shown.

Fix the ETT in place with commercial apparatus (or tape, if short-term intubation is expected)

Practicality: Inexpensive, portable, and simple
　　　　Direct laryngoscopy is the most familiar form of definitive airway management for the majority of practitioners
　　　　While not complex, much practice and experience is required to attain expertise

Indications: Airway patency and/or protection
　　　　Failure of oxygenation
　　　　Failure of ventilation
　　　　Secretion control/suctioning

Manipulation of pH (as in elevated intracranial pressure)
Drug administration (when vascular access is not obtainable during resuscitation)

Contraindications: Laryngeal injury/trauma
　　　　Inaccessibility of oral cavity
　　　　Potential cervical spine trauma (sniffing position and head extension should be avoided; if direct laryngoscopy is chosen as the means of intubation, in-line immobilization of the cervical spine should be utilized)

Complications: Corneal abrasion
Oral and pharyngeal trauma (dental injury, lacerations, sore throat)
Laryngeal trauma (cord avulsion, arytenoids dislocation, hoarseness)
Misplaced ETT, with failure to oxygenate and ventilate
Regurgitation
Aspiration of gastric contents
Endobronchial intubation (usually right mainstem)
Barotrauma (from excessive positive pressure during ventilation)
Bronchospasm
Excessive sympathetic response to intubation (tachycardia, hypertension, dysrhythmias, myocardial ischemia)
Complications of long-term intubation (tracheal stenosis, mouth ulceration)
Neural injury, from traction or pressure (recurrent laryngeal, hypoglossal, or glossopharyngeal nerves)

REFERENCES:

1. Adnet F, Bonon SW, Dumas JL, et al. Study of the "sniffing position" by magnetic resonance imaging. *Anesthesiology* 2001;94:83–86.
2. Adnet F. Common practices and concepts in anesthesia: time for reassessment. *Anesthesiology* 2001;95:825–827.
3. Levitan R, Mechem CC, Ochroch EA, et al. Head elevated laryngoscopy position: improving laryngeal exposure during laryngoscopy by increasing head elevation. *Ann Emerg Med* 2003;41:322–330.
4. Schmitt HJ, Mang H. Head and neck elevation beyond the sniffing position improves laryngeal view in cases of difficult direct laryngoscopy. *J Clin Anesth* 2002;14:335–338.
5. Benumof JL. Difficult laryngoscopy: obtaining the best view. *Can J Anaesth* 1994;41:361–365.
6. Henderson JJ. The use of paraglossal straight blade laryngoscopy in difficult tracheal intubation. *Anaesthesia* 1997;52:552–560.
7. Knill RL. Direct laryngoscopy made easy with a "BURP." *Can J Anaesth* 1993;40:279–282.
8. Benumof JL, Cooper SL. Quantitative improvement in laryngoscopic view by optimal external laryngeal pressure. *J Clin Anesth* 1996;8:136–140.
9. Finucane BT, Santora AH. *Principles of airway management,* 2nd ed. St. Louis: Mosby; 1999:227–250.

4

The Pediatric Airway

Children present unique problems in airway management. By age 8, the anatomy and physiology of the pediatric respiratory system are similar to those of adults. In younger children, the high metabolic rate and body surface area (compared with body mass) result in increased oxygen utilization rates. These rates, coupled with a relatively low functional residual capacity in the unconscious or anesthetized child, predispose younger children to relatively rapid oxygen desaturation. A selection of equipment for pediatric airway management is shown in Figure 4.1.

The anatomy of the pediatric airway differs from that of adults in several particulars. Because of a prominent occiput, infants and small children, when lying supine, tend towards neck flexion, and thus the "sniffing" position recommended in adults is not necessary. A small head ring or "doughnut" to stabilize the head may be beneficial. The tongue is proportionally large in small children, and has a propensity to obstruct ventilation, as does the hypertrophied tonsillar tissue (Fig. 4.2). The nares are small in infants, and adenoidal tissue often partially obstructs the nasopharynx. Nasal airways are seldom used during mask ventilation, in order to avoid epistaxis and injury to the adenoidal tonsils, but correctly sized oral airways are frequently useful. Due to the distensibility and pliability of soft tissues and cartilages of children, it is relatively easy to compress the airway during mask ventilation. For this reason, the practitioner should be careful to confine his/her fingers to the boney mandible during mask ventilation.

The larynx tends to lie higher in the pediatric neck, at the C4 level, as opposed to the C6 level in adults. The epiglottis is longer and inclined toward the glottic opening (Fig. 4.3), which can make it more difficult to elevate during laryngoscopy, particularly with a curved blade. For this reason, straight blades are preferentially used in infants and toddlers. After age 2, airway management is more amenable to the use of curved blades. Because the cricoid cartilage is the narrowest portion of the pediatric airway, and tight seals with inflated cuffs may contribute to mucosal injury with edema, uncuffed tubes have been the mainstay of tracheal intubation in young children. However, cuffed tubes may be used safely, if tight seals are

avoided. Ideally, a small leak should be detected when 20 cm H_2O of airway pressure is applied. Endotracheal tubes (ETT) in children can be chosen to correspond to the size of the small finger, or, more quantitatively, with the following equation:

$$\frac{Age + 16}{4} = ETT \text{ size (internal diameter)}$$

The trachea is relatively short in young children, measuring only 5 cm at birth. It is relatively easy to intubate the mainstem bronchus, and therefore one should be mindful of appropriate endotracheal tube lengths for different pediatric age groups. One equation that helps predict these lengths for orotracheal intubation is:

$$\frac{Age + 12}{2} = \text{Appropriate depth of ETT insertion (in cm)}$$

During mask ventilation of a pediatric patient (Fig. 4.4), airway obstruction is common. Oral airways and a tight-fitting mask, along with appropriate hand position on the mask and jaw usually overcome this readily. In light planes of unconsciousness, laryngospasm is a frequent occurrence in infants and small children (Fig. 4.3). This is best managed with positive pressure by face mask, while a triple airway maneuver is performed. If it proves refractory, a small dose of succinylcholine (0.15 mg/kg) is usually effective in allowing mask ventilation until the process resolves. When all else fails, emergent induction, muscle relaxation with full-dose succinylcholine, and reintubation are necessary.

When direct laryngoscopy is attempted in infants and toddlers, the larynx often appears quite anterior. Attention should be paid to placing the head in extension (extreme cervical flexion causes obstruction, and may worsen the view) and keeping the large tongue displaced to the left, out of the field of vision (Fig. 4.5). External laryngeal pressure, applied by the fingers of the right hand, or even the small finger of the left hand during laryngoscopy, can improve the laryngoscopic grade. Loose deciduous teeth are common, and if possible, their existence should be noted before the procedure (Fig. 4.6).

Figure 4.1 Pediatric airway equipment.

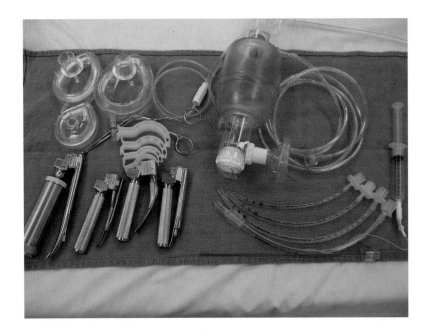

Figure 4.2 Palatine tonsillary hypertrophy in a 6-year-old child.

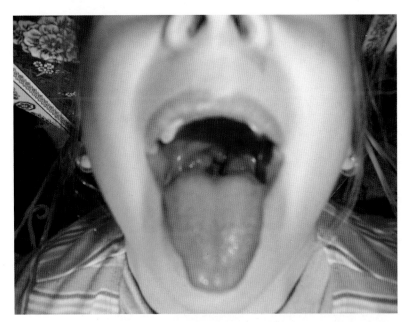

Figure 4.3 The epiglottis of an infant; note cord apposition secondary to laryngospasm in right-hand image. (From Benjamin B, Bingham B, Hawke M, et al. *A color atlas of otorhinolaryngology*. London: Martin Dunitz; 1995, with permission.)

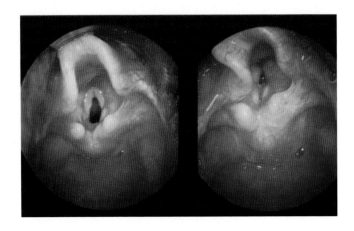

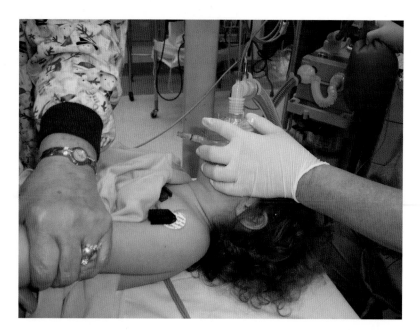

Figure 4.4 Face mask ventilation in a child, showing appropriate placement of the fingers on the ramus of the mandible.

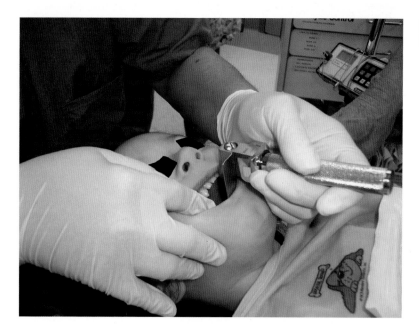

Figure 4.5 Direct laryngoscopy with a MacIntosh blade in a pediatric patient.

Very loose teeth should be extracted after loss of consciousness, to avoid displacement into the airway during laryngoscopy. Confirmation of tube position is similar to that in adults, with special attention paid to the depth of the ETT in the trachea. Once established as appropriate, this should be noted, since even small degrees of cervical flexion or extension can result in 2 cm to 3 cm of ETT motion, with endobronchial intubation an ever-present danger.

For small children, a form of the T-piece circuit is usually used for ventilation during anesthesia, due to its light weight, portability, and low resistance to spontaneous ventilation. When a bag is incorporated into the circuit, it is referred to as a Jackson-Rees modification. These circuits require a fresh gas flow of at least 2.5 times the child's minute ventilation to avoid rebreathing of carbon dioxide. During intubation or resuscitation outside the operating room, a suitably-sized self-inflating ventilation bag is utilized, with high-flow oxygen.

When intubation fails, many of the tools and techniques discussed elsewhere in this book can be utilized for pediatric patients. These include airway stylets, digital intubation, laryngeal mask airways (LMA), and fiberoptic and rigid scopes (the Bullard laryngoscope is made in a

Figure 4.6 Missing deciduous teeth in a 7-year-old child.

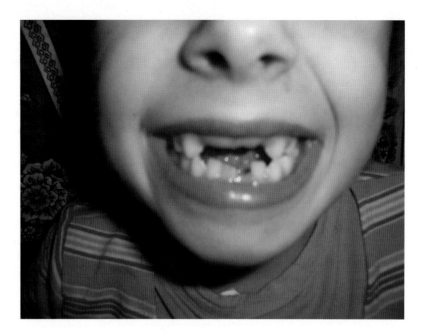

pediatric size, as are many fiberscopes). However, some of the choices available for adults are not readily utilized in children. Awake, blind nasotracheal intubation is not likely to be tolerated by a child, and the nasal obstruction offered by adenoidal tonsils makes epistaxis more likely than in the adult. Some devices, such as the intubating LMA, are not available in pediatric sizes. The cricothyroid membrane is so small in infants and toddlers as to be virtually inaccessible. In older children, up to age 8, needle cricothyrotomy with transtracheal jet ventilation is usually possible, but formal surgical cricothyrotomy is difficult.

REFERENCES:

1. Steward DJ. *Manual of pediatric anesthesia*, 4th ed. New York: Churchill-Livingstone; 1995:15–16,80–85.
2. Riazi J. The difficult pediatric airway. In: Benumof JL, ed. *Airway management, principles and practice*. St. Louis: Mosby; 1996:585–596.
3. Finucane BT, Santora AH. *Principles of airway management*, 2nd ed. St. Louis: Mosby; 1996:285–313.
4. Luten RC, Kissoon N. Approach to the pediatric airway. In: Walls RM, Murphy MF, Luten RC, et al, eds. *Manual of emergency airway management*, 2nd ed. Philadelphia: Lippincott Williams & Wilkins; 2004:212–220.

5

Confirmation of Endotracheal Tube Placement

Misplaced endotracheal tubes (ETT) can result in severe morbidity and mortality. As soon as an ETT is inserted, its presence in the trachea must be confirmed. No simple, foolproof test exists that incontrovertibly establishes that the tube is situated in the airway. Confirmation is best carried out with a combination of CO_2 detection and physical examination maneuvers. Detection of exhaled CO_2 is widely accepted as the most reliable, readily available method of confirming ETT placement. This is accomplished in the operating room with capnography (continuous monitoring of end-tidal CO_2, displayed graphically on a dedicated monitor) (Fig. 5.1A), and in most emergency intubations with a color-change indicator (a purple-to-yellow change indicates presence of greater than 4% CO in exhaled gases) (Fig. 5.1B,C). While CO_2 detection reliably localizes the tube in the airway, it does not distinguish between tracheal and endobronchial intubation. Furthermore, both false positive and false negative results may occur (1). When cardiac arrest occurs, or blood flow through the lungs is markedly diminished, exhaled CO_2 will be near zero, even when the tube is correctly placed. Other methods of confirmation are preferred under these circumstances. On the other hand, during esophageal intubation, CO_2 may be detected from the gases insufflated into the stomach during mask ventilation. This usually rapidly diminishes over four to five breaths. If end-tidal CO_2 is detectable and stable (not diminishing) thereafter, the tube is almost certainly in the airway (2).

When no means of CO_2 detection is available, or cardiac arrest occurs, the esophageal bulb detector device provides a means to ascertain whether the tube is in the airway or the esophagus (Fig. 5.2A,B). Since the trachea (and bronchi) possess cartilaginous walls, and contain a column of air, a collapsed bulb device attached to the proximal end of an ETT in the airway should suction air and rapidly reinflate. On the other hand, if an ETT is placed in the esophagus, the deflated bulb applies suction to the tube that results in apposition of the mucous membranes to the distal orifice of the tube, preventing bulb reinflation (3).

Physical exam maneuvers complement the above methods of ETT confirmation (Figs. 5.3 and 5.4). These include chest auscultation (which should be carried out in the axillae) (Fig. 5.4), evidence of chest rise, absence of gastric distension or sounds of gastric insufflation, the presence of vapor in the ETT tube during apparent exhalation and "balloting" of the ETT cuff above the sternal notch while palpating the pilot tube (4) (Fig. 5.3). None of these methods is entirely reliable, but in combination with CO_2 detection (or the esophageal bulb detector, if CO_2 is not likely to be present) they should nearly eliminate the possibility of esophageal intubation.

Chest radiography likewise can contribute to tube localization. However, the lateral x-ray is considerably more reliable in this regard than an anterior-posterior film, since superimposition of an esophageal ETT over the trachea can be misleading. Although frequently unavailable outside of the operating room or critical care unit, fiberoptic bronchoscopy is a highly accurate method to ascertain correct tube position (5), as it provides direct visualization of the ETT and its location.

Figure 5.1 A. Capnography in the operating room. B. CO_2 color-change indicator: purple color before connection to circuit. C. The indicator turns yellow when connected to the circuit, indicating correct ETT placement.

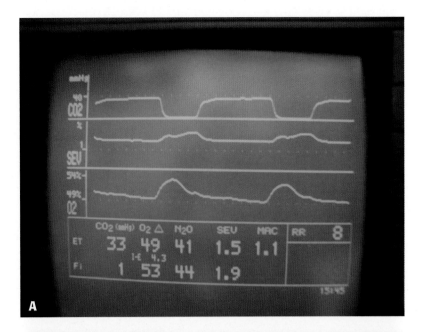

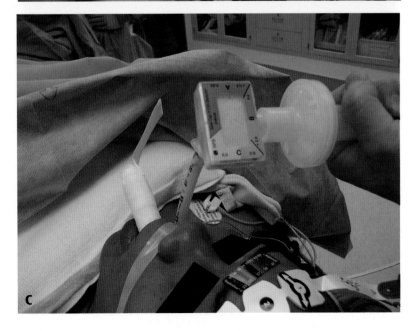

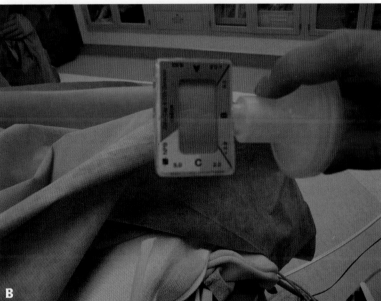

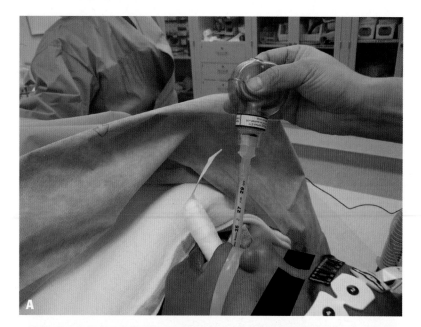

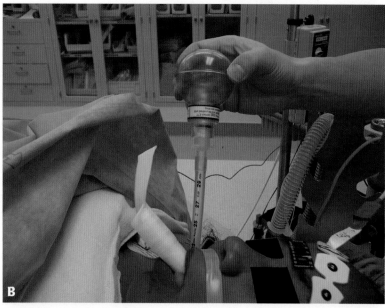

Figure 5.2 A. An esophageal bulb detector device. **B.** When placed on the end of the ETT, and deflated, it should reinflate if the ETT is in the trachea.

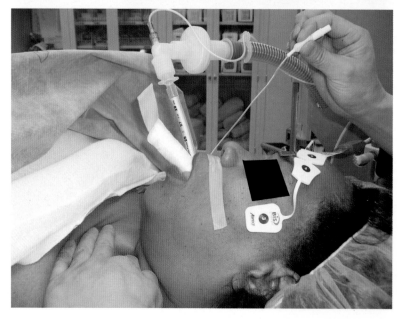

Figure 5.3 "Balloting" the ETT cuff in the trachea while palpating the pilot tube.

Figure 5.4 Auscultation in the axillary area contributes to confirmation of ETT placement.

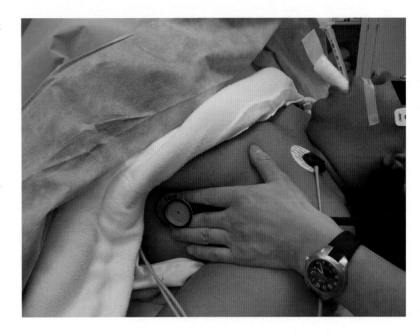

REFERENCES:

1. Andersen KH, Hald A. Assessing the position of the tracheal tube: the reliability of different methods. *Anaesthesia* 1989;44:984–990.

2. Birmingham PK, Cheney FW, Ward RJ. Esophageal intubation: a review of detection techniques. *Anesth Analg* 1986;65:886–896.

3. Zaleski L, Abello D, Gold MI. The esophageal detector device. Does it work? *Anesthesiology* 1993;79:244–251.

4. Salem MR, Baraka A. Confirmation of tracheal intubation. In: Benumof JL, ed. *Airway management, principles and practice.* St. Louis: Mosby; 1996: 531–560.

5. Benumof JL. Management of the difficult adult airway: with special emphasis on awake tracheal intubation. *Anesthesiology* 1991;75:1087–1110.

6

Retraction Blades for Direct Laryngoscopy

As noted in the prior chapter, the purpose of a laryngoscope is to retract the mandible and the soft tissues of the mouth and anterior oropharynx upwards, allowing exposure of the glottis. In cross section, the blade of the laryngoscope typically consists of a flat portion, or spatula, and a vertical portion, or flange, along with a light source. These components have been arrayed in a large variety of shapes and configurations to meet the challenge of elevating soft tissues during retraction and keeping them out of the line of sight of the laryngoscopist, while permitting the necessary manipulations to insert an endotracheal tube (ETT). Since the origins of laryngoscopy, in the late 19th century, laryngoscopes have undergone an evolution in shape. Early versions had a "C" shape configuration, but did not have either detachable blades or an intrinsic light source. By the middle of the 20th century, laryngoscopes had been developed that had detachable blades and built-in light sources. More modern laryngoscopes contain a light source in the handle with fiberoptic bundles in the blades. The older-style laryngoscopes remain in use by ear-nose-throat (ENT) surgeons today for diagnostic and therapeutic procedures involving the airway.

Many different types of retraction blades for direct laryngoscopy are available today. Although many variations of the straight and curved blade exist, the Miller and MacIntosh blades, introduced about 60 years ago, remain preeminent (1,2). Conventionally, the straight blade is inserted beneath the epiglottis and used to directly expose the glottis. The curved blade fits into the vallecula, exerting upward traction on the glossoepiglottic ligament as it is lifted, to flip the epiglottis superiorly, allowing the operator to see the exposed glottis (Figs. 6.1 to 6.4). Certain situations, such as a very "deep" glottis, or protuberant "buck" incisor teeth, favor use of the straight blade. Some variants of the Miller blade, such as the Phillips blade (Fig. 6.1), or the Wisconsin blade, have a higher vertical profile, answering one of the deficiencies of this type of blade: inadequate space for endotracheal tube manipulation in the pharynx, despite an adequate view of the glottis. Other varieties of laryngoscope blade that may prove useful in unusual situations include angled blades and blades with no vertical flange (Fig. 6.5). These are not commonly used in clinical practice. Table 6.1 details characteristics of some unusual blades.

The McCoy laryngoscope blade is an articulating blade that allows one to lift its distal tip in order to improve the view of the glottis, if the epiglottis remains downfolded and impedes visibility (3). This blade has been compared to the standard MacIntosh blade, and potentially can improve the laryngoscopic view, but does not do so consistently (4,5). A double-angle blade has been developed that combines features of both the straight and curved laryngoscope blade (6) (Fig. 6.6). The "Improved View MacIntosh" blade allows an enhanced view of the larynx, due to a concavity in the flat portion of the blade (7) (Fig. 6.7).

Figure 6.1 Miller and Phillips laryngoscope blades.

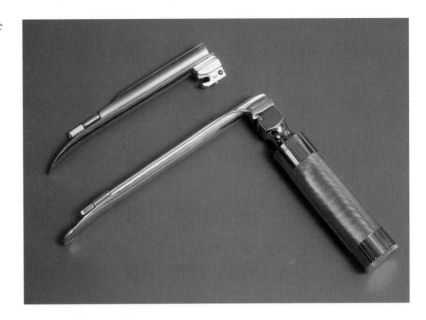

Figure 6.2 Miller blade shown lifting epiglottis to expose glottis.

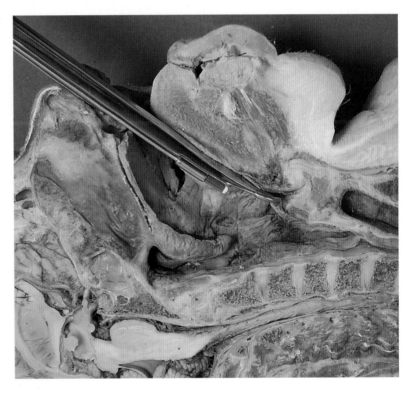

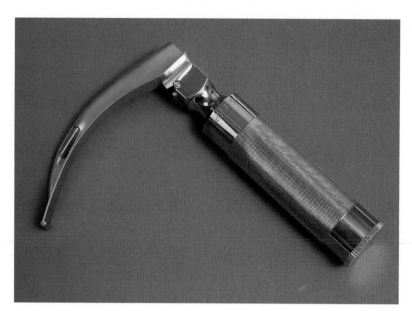

Figure 6.3 MacIntosh laryngoscope blade.

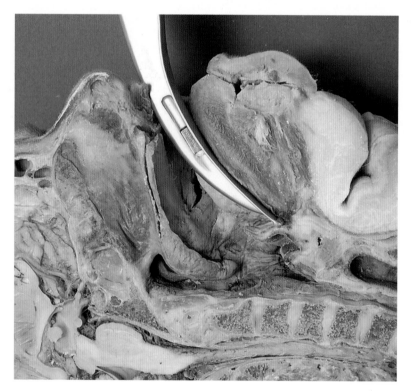

Figure 6.4 MacIntosh blade shown with tip in vallecula.

Figure 6.5 Bizzari-Giuffrida laryngoscope blade: no vertical flange is present, to allow insertion into small oral cavity or those patients who cannot open the mouth well.

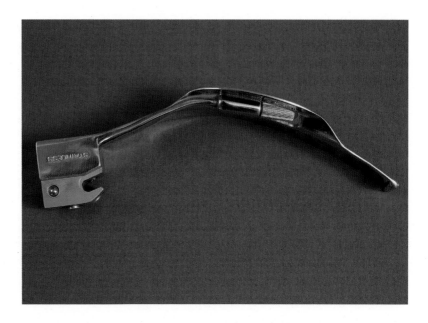

Table 6.1

Selected Retraction Blades

Blade	Characteristics	Uses/Advantages
Miller	Straight with curved tip	Normal airway, long epiglottis, "deep" glottis, prominent upper incisors
Phillips, Wisconsin	Straight blades with higher vertical profiles	More room for ETT placement than Miller blade
MacIntosh	Curved blade	Normal airway
Bizzarri-Giuffrida	Curved blade with no vertical flange	For small mouth or protruding or fragile teeth
Siker	Incorporates mirror into blade	For anterior-situated larynx
Choi	Has double-angle shape	Better exposure of anterior larynx
Belscope	Angulated, with optional prism attachment	For normal airway, or anterior larynx
McCoy	Version of MacIntosh blade with articulated tip	Facilitates lifting of epiglottis
Improved-View MacIntosh	Concavity in long axis of spatula	Provides better view of anterior larynx

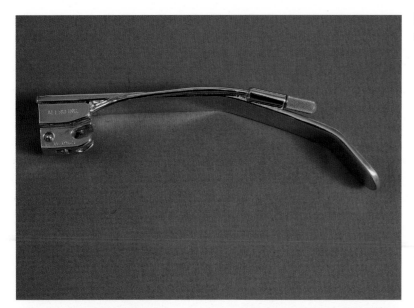

Figure 6.6 Choi (double angle) laryngoscope blade.

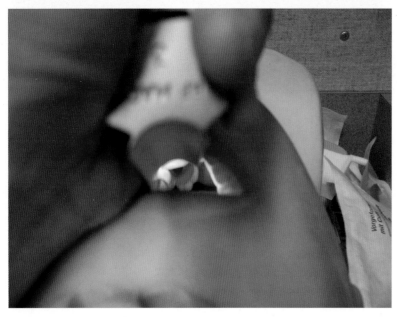

Figure 6.7 "Improved View" MacIntosh laryngoscope blade. This blade contains a concavity in the flat portion or "spoon" of the blade, permitting a better view of the glottis.

REFERENCES:

1. Miller RA. A new laryngoscope. *Anesthesiology* 1941;1: 317–319.
2. MacIntosh RR. A new laryngoscope. *Lancet* 1943;1:205.
3. McCoy ED, Mirakhur RK. The levering laryngoscope. *Anaesth* 1993;48:516–518.
4. Cook TM, Tuckey JP. A comparison between the MacIntosh and McCoy laryngoscope blades. *Anaesth* 1996;51:977–980.
5. Tuckey JP, Cook TM. An evaluation of the levering laryngoscope. *Anaesth* 1996;51:71–73.
6. Choi JJ. An angulated laryngoscope for routine and difficult tracheal intubation. *Anesthesiology* 1990;72:576.
7. Racz GB. Improved vision modification of the MacIntosh Laryngoscope (letter) *Anaesth* 1984;39:1249.

Pharmacology of Airway Management

For most patients, endotracheal intubation, or placement of a supraglottic ventilation device such as the laryngeal mask airway, is uncomfortable and frightening, even intolerable. Pharmacologic tools for managing anxiety, and controlling the level of consciousness and muscle activity are therefore essential. However, in some circumstances, airway management is best conducted without rendering a patient unconscious, apneic, or paralyzed. Such situations include upper airway foreign bodies or airway obstruction, severe facial trauma with unrecognizable anatomy, and prediction of difficult or impossible laryngoscopy (especially if face mask ventilation appears likely to be difficult as well). Under such conditions, use of drugs that make the patient apneic, combined with an inability to intubate and/or ventilate, becomes life-threatening (see section II, Difficult Airway Management). Therefore such patients are best dealt with by utilizing an awake approach to management of the airway. They may benefit from modest amounts of sedation to facilitate this, titrated to allay anxiety and reduce discomfort while avoiding respiratory failure. For this purpose, a combination of a benzodiazepine and an opioid are commonly selected (Table 7.1).

For patients in shock, those already unconscious, and those in extremus, such sedation is either unnecessary or impractical due to time constraints. Even small doses of sedative and opioid drugs can cause significant respiratory depression and worsen already compromised hemodynamics. Topical anesthesia of the oral, pharyngeal and airway mucosa, nerve blocks of the upper airway, and/or subcutaneous local anesthesia injection over the larynx to prepare for needle insertion or incision, should be utilized for awake techniques if time permits, in order to improve patient tolerance and reduce the hemodynamic response to intubation (see Chapter 20).

For most cases requiring intubation, including emergent airway management in the emergency department and elsewhere, patients are rendered unconscious for the procedure (1,2). Induction of anesthesia along with provision of muscle relaxation provides optimum intubating conditions and the best opportunity for visualization of the glottis with direct laryngoscopy (3). For routine cases in euvolemic patients, sodium thiopental or propofol are appropriate induction agents, while etomidate is preferred for those with uncertain volume status, recent trauma, or evidence of hypovolemia (4) (Table 7.2). When patients present in frank shock, or with unstable hemodynamics, ketamine is favored for induction, due to its sympathomimetic properties.

After the hypnotic is administered, a muscle relaxant is delivered, typically the depolarizing agent succinylcholine, for adult elective cases (Table 7.3). This agent is favored for its rapid onset (45 seconds) and relatively brief duration of action (6 to 8 minutes) (5). The drug has numerous undesirable side effects and adverse reactions, however, and its pharmacology must be well understood for its safe use (Table 7.4)(6). Because of its adverse effects on children with unrecognized myopathies, succinylcholine is avoided in elective, pediatric anesthesia cases, but may be utilized in children for emergent intubation (7). In general, use of muscle relaxants to facilitate endotracheal intubation should be undertaken only by physicians (or nurse anesthetists) with considerable experience and skill in management of the airway, as prolonged apnea will quickly occur after administration. Furthermore, they should not be used without due consideration of the fact that they provide only muscle paralysis, and do not address the patient's level of consciousness or perception. During emergency intubation, succinylcholine is frequently chosen due to its rapid onset time. When succinylcholine is contraindicated, several nondepolarizing relaxants can be utilized to provide relaxation (Table 7.3). The drug in this class with an onset profile closest to that of succinylcholine is rocuronium, which provides good intubating conditions in about 60 seconds.

In the fasted, elective surgery patient, with little risk of regurgitation or passive reflux during airway management, induction is followed by face mask ventilation as the muscle relaxant is administered and its onset awaited. This serves to maintain oxygenation during the apneic period, as well as to provide the intubator with a sense of confidence that, should endotracheal tube placement fail, the patient can be managed with face mask ventilation while assistance is obtained.

In cases of emergent airway management, however, and whenever there is risk of vomiting or passive regurgitation after airway reflexes are lost (patients with full stomach, uncertain gastric contents, or a history of reflux or swallowing disorders), the threat of aspiration of gastric contents is significant. For this reason, a rapid sequence induction, termed "rapid sequence intubation" in emer-

Table 7.1

Agents Utilized for Preoperative or Preprocedural Sedation/Analgesia in Adults

Agent	Dose	Effect
Midazolam	0.5 mg to 2 mg IV	Sedation/amnesia
Diazepam	2.5 mg to 5 mg IV	Sedation/amnesia
Fentanyl	25 µg to 100 µg IV	Analgesia
Morphine	2.5 mg to 5 mg IV	Analgesia

gency intubation outside the operating room (OR), should be carried out. The hypnotic agent and muscle relaxant are injected intravenously in rapid succession, without attempts at ventilation between administration of the two, and face mask ventilation is withheld unless oxygen desaturation occurs. In order to minimize the period of apnea during rapid sequence induction, succinylcholine or rocuronium are utilized for muscle relaxation. Before consciousness and airway reflexes are lost, cricoid pressure is initiated by an assistant to reduce the likelihood of gastric reflux and aspiration, and is continued until the endotracheal tube has been placed and its position in the airway confirmed. After waiting the appropriate period for muscle relaxation, direct laryngoscopy is carried out and the endotracheal tube placed. After its position in the trachea is ascertained, it is secured, and ventilation initiated, completing the rapid sequence technique.

In some circumstances, premedication before rapid sequence induction may serve to reduce adverse responses to drugs or the physical manipulations of the airway. These include administration of lidocaine to blunt the impact of intubation on elevated intracranial pressure, opioids to reduce the hemodynamic response to laryngoscopy and intubation, or pretreatment with a small dose of a nondepolarizing neuromuscular blocking agent to reduce muscle fasciculations from succinylcholine (and the atten-

dant elevations in intraocular or intragastric pressure that may occur as a result of these fasciculations).

Induction Sequence for Elective Anesthesia with Endotracheal Intubation:

Preparations for direct laryngoscopy (Chapter 3)
Pre-induction sedation, if required
Placement of patient monitors
Assurance of adequate suction and reliable intravenous access
Pre-oxygenation with well-fit face mask
Administration of hypnotic agent
Mask ventilation
Administration of muscle relaxant
Continue mask ventilation
Direct laryngoscopy
Endotracheal tube placement
Confirmation of tube location in trachea
Fixation of endotracheal tube

Induction Sequence for Rapid Sequence Induction (Rapid Sequence Intubation):

Preparations for direct laryngoscopy (see Chapter 3)
Placement of patient monitors
Assurance of adequate suction and reliable intravenous access
Place stylet in endotracheal tube
Pre-oxygenation
Provision of cricoid pressure by assistant
Administration of hypnotic agent (usually propofol or thiopental in OR; most commonly etomidate in the emergency department or other emergent settings)
Administration of muscle relaxant (succinylcholine or rocuronium)
Direct laryngoscopy
Endotracheal tube placement
Confirmation of tube location in trachea
Release of cricoid pressure
Fixation of endotracheal tube

Table 7.2

Agents Utilized for Routine and Rapid Sequence Induction of Anesthesia

Agent	IV Dose (mg/kg)	Time to Onset (s)	Expected Duration of Action After Induction Dose (min)
Propofol	Adults: 2.0–2.5 Pediatric: 2.5–3.5	30	5–10
Sodium Thiopental	Adults: 3.0–5.0 Pediatrics: 4.0–7.0	30	5–10
Etomidate	Adults: 0.25–0.3 Pediatrics: 0.3–0.4	15–45	3–12
Ketamine	Adults: 1.0–3.0 Pediatrics: 2.0–4.0	45–60	10–20

Table 7.3

Neuromuscular Relaxants for Endotracheal Intubation

Drug	Category	Intubating Dose (IV)	Time of Onset (s)	Duration (min)
Succinylcholine	Depolarizing agent	Adult: 1.5 mg/kg Pediatric: 2.0 mg/kg*	45 45	7–8 7–8
Mivacurium	Short-acting, nondepolarizing	0.2 mg/kg	2–2.5	15–20
Vecuronium	Intermediate-acting, nondepolarizing	0.1 mg/kg	2.5–3	30–45
Rocuronium	Intermediate-acting, nondepolarizing	0.6–1.2 mg/kg	1 min (with higher dose)	30–45

*Succinylcholine is usually administered with atropine, 10–20 mg/kg, in infants and young children, in whom bradycardia is a common response to this agent.

Table 7.4

Adverse Responses and Contraindications to Succinylcholine

Adverse Responses	Contraindications
Muscle fasciculation	Known sensitivity or allergy
Muscle soreness	History of, or risk of, MH
Hypertonicity of masseter muscles	Hyperkalemia
Hyperkalemia/dysrhythmia/cardiac arrest	Myopathy or muscular dystrophy
Increased intraocular pressure	Lower motor neuron paralysis*
Increased intragastric pressure	Upper motor neuron paralysis*
Increased intracranial pressure	Major burn*
Allergic reaction (hives, anaphylaxis)	Pseudocholinesterase deficiency
Triggering of MH	
Prolonged blockade (Phase 2 block)	
Inability to metabolize with prolonged blockade (Pseudocholinesterase deficiency)	
Bradycardia	
Dysrhythmias	

*Risk is increased more than 24 hours after the acute insult. MH, malignant hyperthermia.

REFERENCES:

1. Walls RM, Gurr DE, Kulkarni RG, et al. 6294 Emergency department intubations: second report of the ongoing National Emergency Airway Registry (NEAR) II study. *Ann Emerg Med* 2000;36:S51.

2. Sakles JC, Laurin EG, Rantapaa AA, et al. Airway management in the emergency department: a one-year study of 610 tracheal intubations. *Ann Emerg Med* 1998;31:325–332.

3. Benumof JL. Difficult laryngoscopy: obtaining the best view. *Can J Anaesth* 1994;41:361–365.

4. Chiu JW, White PF. Nonopioid intravenous anesthesia. In: Barish PG, Cullen BF, Stoelting RK, eds. *Clinical anesthesia*, 4th ed. Philadelphia: Lippincott William & Wilkins; 2001: 327–343.

5. White PF. *Anesthesia drug manual*. Philadelphia: W.B. Saunders; 1996:300.

6. Orebaugh SL. Succinylcholine: Adverse effects and alternatives in emergency medicine. *Am J Emerg Med* 1999;17: 715–721.

7. Cravero JP, Rice LJ. Pediatric anesthesia. In: Barish PG, Cullen BF, Stoelting RK, eds. *Clinical anesthesia*, 4th ed. Philadelphia: Lippincott William & Wilkins; 2001:1195–1204.

Definitions, Incidence, and Predictors of the Difficult Airway

The term "difficult airway" defies simple definition. It may be interpreted to mean that laryngoscopy reveals a poor view of the airway, that endotracheal tube placement is impossible, or that mask ventilation is not feasible. Some of these ideas have been expressed quantitatively: difficult mask ventilation is defined by the American Society of Anesthesiology as the inability of a trained anesthetist to maintain a patient's oxygen saturation above 90% by using face mask ventilation (assuming a normal saturation at baseline), whereas difficult intubation is defined as an inability to place an endotracheal tube within 10 minutes or three attempts at direct laryngoscopy (1).

Difficult intubation usually corresponds to poor glottic visualization during direct laryngoscopy, or a high-grade laryngeal view with inability to see the vocal cords or even part of the glottic aperture (2). The standard classification for grading the laryngeal view at direct laryngoscopy derives from Cormack and Lehane (Fig. 8.1) (3), who proposed a four-grade scheme which facilitates communication between practitioners as well as investigators. Grade 1 corresponds to a view of the entire glottic opening; grade 2 to a view in which only a portion of the opening is visible; grade 3 to the visualization of only the arytenoids or the epiglottis; and grade 4 to an inability to see the glottis or epiglottis at all (Figs. 8.2 to 8.5). Most patients have anatomy which allows grade 1 or grade 2 views, with uncomplicated intubation, while a small minority present grade 3 or grade 4 views, which can be quite challenging or preclude intubation with direct laryngoscopy altogether.

Difficulty with glottic exposure during laryngoscopy also can be quantitated by the "percent of glottic opening" score, which corresponds to the proportion of the opening that can be visualized (4). Adnet et al developed an "intubation difficulty scale," which has been validated prospectively, and which corresponds well to the time required for intubation, and to a visual analog scale assessment of procedural difficulty by those carrying out intubation (5).

Many investigators have set out to document the incidence of difficult airways in the perioperative setting. Grade 3 laryngoscopic views, requiring multiple attempts at intubation, occur in 1% to 13% of all patients presenting for surgery (6–9). Severe grade 3 to grade 4 views, making

intubation extremely difficult, are estimated to occur in 0.05% to 0.9% of general anesthesia cases, but is more rare in populations with normal cervical mobility (7,10–12). Difficult mask ventilation presents in 2.4% to 5% of such cases (13,14). Fortunately, the simultaneous occurrence of both inability to intubate and inability to ventilate by face mask is quite rare, on the order of 2 in 10,000 cases (15,16). However, mild difficulty with intubation requiring a change of blades and/or laryngoscopists in the operating room is fairly common, with an incidence ranging from 1% to18% (16–18).

The incidence of difficult airways in the emergency department populations has not been studied as thoroughly as that in the operating room. Sakles et al described intubation in 610 patients in an urban emergency department (ED) over a one-year period, 84% of whom were managed with the rapid sequence intubation (RSI) technique. The success rate of these intubations was 99%, with 1% of patients requiring emergent surgical airway (19). Esophageal intubation occurred initially in 5% of patients, with rapid correction. Thus, it appears that 6% of patients presented some difficulty in airway management to the emergency physicians involved. Overall, 5% required three or more attempts at laryngoscopy, so that the range of difficult airways appears to be between 6% and 11%, depending on whether these latter categories overlapped. However, another 16% of patients were deemed unfit for RSI. In the investigation of Tayal et al, the proportion of patients whom the investigators were unable to manage with direct laryngoscopy was likewise low, as only 1% required a surgical airway (20). However, 30% of patients who were intubated were not included in the analysis because they did not meet the investigators' requirements for eligibility for RSI. Thus, the actual incidence of difficult airways lies somewhere between the extremes of 1% and 30%. Even if the lower range is chosen, difficult airways in the ED are not rare, and appear to be more common than in the population presenting for elective surgery. In a recent multicenter study of ED airway management in more than 6,300 cases, the incidence of esophageal intubation was found to be 4%, and the failure rate for intubation when RSI was utilized to secure the airway was less than 2% (21,22).

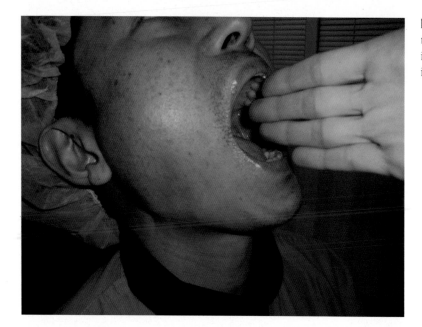

Figure 8.11 Normal range of motion of the temporomandibular joint should permit insertion of three fingers aligned vertically into the patient's mouth.

milieu of the emergency department, the intensive care unit, or the hospital floors. The utility of these predictors in the emergency setting has not been demonstrated, and indeed, they may not be practical for many patients who present to the emergency department, due to altered mental status, lack of cooperation, or cervical spine protection measures (32). Nevertheless, when time and circumstances permit, a rapid assessment of mouth opening, tongue size, cervical mobility, and thyromental distance may help the physician avoid a disastrous sequence of events, by helping to predict which patients may not be managed successfully with bag-mask ventilation and/or intubation after rendered unconscious and apneic.

REFERENCES:

1. ASA Practice guidelines for the management of the difficult airway. *Anesthesiology* 1993;78:597–600.
2. Benumof JL. Management of the difficult airway. *Anesthesiology* 1991;75:1087–1110.
3. Cormack RS, Lehane J. Difficult tracheal intubation in obstetrics. *Anaesthesia* 1984;39:1105–1111.
4. Levitan R, Ochtroch EA, Kush S. Validation of the Percentage of Glottic Opening (POGO) score. *Acad Emerg Med* 1998;5:482.
5. Adnet F, Borron SW, Racine SX, et al. The intubation difficulty scale (IDS). *Anesthesiology* 1997;87:1273–1274.
6. Wilson ME, Spiegelhalter D, Robertson JA, et al. Predicting difficult intubation. *Br J Anaesth* 1988;61:211–216.
7. Williams KN, Carli F, Cormack RS. Unexpected difficult laryngoscopy. *Br J Anaesth* 1991;66:38–44.
8. Cohen SM, Laurito C, Segil LJ. Oral exam to predict difficult intubation. *Anesthesiology* 1989;71:A937.
9. Tse JC, Rimm EB, Hussain A. Predicting difficult endotracheal intuition in surgical patients scheduled for general anesthesia: a prospective blind study. *Anesth Analg* 1995;81:254–258.
10. Samsoon GLT, Young JRB. Difficult tracheal intubation. *Anaesth* 1987;42:487–490.
11. Glassenberg R, Vaisrub N, Albright G. Incidence of failed intubation in obstetrics. *Anesthesiology* 1991;73:A1061.
12. Combes X, Le Roux B, Suen P, et al. Unanticipated difficult airway in anesthetized patients: prospective validation of a management algorithm. *Anesthesiology* 2004;100:1146–1150.
13. Langeron O, Masso E, Huraux C, et al. Prediction of difficult mask ventilation. *Anesthesiology* 2000;92:1229–1236.
14. Cattano D, Panicucci, E, Paolicchi A, et al. Risk factors of the difficult airway: an Italian survey of 1956 patients. *Anesth Analg* 2004;99:1774–1779.
15. Bellhouse CP, Dore C. Criteria for estimating likelihood of endotracheal intubation with MacIntosh laryngoscope. *Anaesth Int Care* 1988;16:329–337.
16. Benumof JL, Scheller MS. Importance of transtracheal jet ventilation in the management of the difficult airway. *Anesthesiology* 1982;71:769–778.
17. Tunstall ME. Failed intubation in the parturient. *Can J Anaesth* 1989;36:611–612.
18. Keenan RL, Bousan CP. Decreasing frequency of anaesthetic cardiac arrest. *J Clin Anesth* 1991;3:354–357.
19. Sakles JC, Laurin EG, Tantapaa AA, et al. Airway management in the emergency department: a one-year study of 610 tracheal intubations. *Ann Emerg Med* 1998;31:325–332.
20. Tayal VS, Riggs RW, Marx JA, et al. Rapid sequence intubation at an emergency medicine residency. *Acad Emerg Med* 1999;6:31–37.
21. Walls RM, Gurr DE, Kulkarni RG, et al. 6294 Emergency department intubations: second report of the Ongoing National Emergency Airway Registry (NEAR) II study. *Ann Emerg Med* 2000;36:S51.
22. Li J. Capnography alone is imperfect for endotracheal tube placement confirmation during emergency intubation. *J Emerg Med* 2001;20:223–239.
23. Dufour DG, Larose DL, Clement SC. Rapid sequence intubation in the emergency department. *J Emerg Med* 1995; 13:705–710.

24. Walls RM. Management of difficult airway in the trauma patient. *Emerg Med Clin North Am* 1998;16:45–61.

25. Nolan JP, Wilson ME. Orotracheal intubation in patients with potential C-spine injuries. *Anesthesiology* 1993;48:630–633.

26. Mallampati SR. Clinical signs to predict difficult tracheal intubation (hypothesis). *Can Anaesth Soc J* 1983;30:316–318.

27. Mallampati SR, Gatt SP, Gugino LD, et al. A clinical sign to predict difficult tracheal intubation: a prospective study. *Can Anaesth Soc J* 1985;32:429–434.

28. Chou HC, Wu TL. Mandibulohyoid distance in difficult laryngoscopy. *Br J Anaesth* 1993;71:335–339.

29. Frerk CM, Till CB, Bradley AJ. Difficult intubation temporomandibular distance and atlanto-occipital gap. *Anaesth* 1996;51:738–740.

30. Watson CB. Prediction of difficult intubation. *Resp Care* 1999;44:777–798.

31. Randell T. Prediction of difficult intubation. *Acta Anaesth Scand* 1996;40:1016–1023.

32. Levitan RM, Everett WW, Ochtroch EA. Limitations of difficult airway prediction in patients intubated in the emergency department. *Ann Emerg Med* 2004;44: 307–313.

9

Decision Making in Difficult Airway Management

Indications for intubation of the trachea vary significantly with different clinical scenarios. In the operating room (OR), this is carried out most frequently to ensure airway patency and protection for the unconscious patient, as well as positive pressure ventilation when muscle paralysis is required for surgery. In the setting of acute respiratory failure or urgent patient resuscitation, the requirements for oxygenation or ventilation usually dominate the decision to intubate. Other indications for intubation include management of secretions, manipulation of cerebral blood flow or serum pH through hyperventilation, and, rarely, administration of drugs via the tracheal route (Table 9.1).

When airway management appears to be challenging, or difficulty is encountered unexpectedly, several guidelines are available to assist the practitioner with decision making. In many cases, difficulty with glottic exposure can be predicted from even a cursory examination of the patient. In others, it is only apparent after a hypnotic and muscle relaxants have been administered, during attempted laryngoscopy. Multiple attempts at direct laryngoscopy may lead to supraglottic swelling and bleeding, deterioration of ventilation, and hypoxemia with potential morbidity (1,2). Because of the potential for morbidity and mortality when airway management fails or is difficult, the American Society of Anesthesiology (ASA) developed the ASA Difficult Airway Algorithm, introduced in 1993, and updated in 2003 (Fig. 9.1) (3,4). Since its implementation in the United States, morbidity, mortality, and claims related to airway management in the OR appear to have fallen significantly (5).

The guideline requires an assessment of those aspects of the airway that are likely to be compromised, if any. Next, one considers how best to approach the patient's airway management: should he or she be intubated awake or after induction of anesthesia? Should spontaneous ventilation be abolished with muscle relaxants, or preserved? Is the airway anatomy or pathology so severe that a surgical approach should be adopted from the beginning? If the airway appears to be difficult to manage, the patient should remain awake with spontaneous ventilation until the endotracheal tube is effectively placed. A number of interventions may be utilized, including retrograde intubation, an "awake look" with direct laryngoscopy after topical anesthesia to the oral mucosa, fiberoptic bronchoscopic intubation (FOB), and placement of a surgical airway under local anesthesia, all of which allow the patient to continue spontaneous ventilation during the intervention.

On the other hand, when difficulty is not predicted in the surgical patient, but is encountered during direct laryngoscopy after induction of anesthesia, the practitioner should immediately call for help, take measures to ensure ongoing ventilation and oxygenation, and consider awakening the patient. Beyond this point, the decision making framework hinges on whether or not bag-mask ventilation is effective after attempts at direct laryngoscopy fail. If so, then a number of options exist, including placing a supraglottic ventilation device, such as the laryngeal mask airway (LMA); allowing the patient to emerge from anesthesia; or utilizing adjuncts to direct laryngoscopy (exotic blades, prisms, mirrors, airway stylets) or other tools to place an endotracheal tube. In addition, a surgical airway under controlled circumstances may be performed. Ongoing ventilation, with preserved oxygenation, allows time for any of these courses to be elected.

However, if bag-mask ventilation is not adequate after attempts at direct laryngoscopy fail in the unconscious, apneic patient, effective ventilation must be instituted immediately (the "emergency pathway"). In the initial algorithm, any of four interventions were considered to be of equal effectiveness: two supraglottic ventilation devices, the LMA and esophageal-tracheal combitube (ETC), and two infraglottic procedures, needle cricothyrotomy (transtracheal "jet" ventilation) and surgical cricothyrotomy (4). When the guidelines were re-released in 2003, favorable experience with the LMA had accrued, and it is now the recommended initial intervention in the emergency pathway (3).

Table 9.1

Indications for Tracheal Intubation

Indication	Example
Airway patency	Unconscious patient
Airway protection	Patient at risk for aspiration
Oxygenation failure	Pneumonia with hypoxemia
Ventilation failure	Severe asthma with respiratory failure
Management of secretions	Copious sputum from pneumonitis
Provision of hyperventilation	Increased intracranial pressure
Drug administration	Inability to secure intravenous access
Muscle paralysis for surgery	Intra-abdominal and intrathoracic surgery

Although the ASA algorithm has proven useful for airway management in surgical cases in the operating room, it has limitations in emergent airway management in other settings. There are significant differences in the nature of airway management and the patient population in the operating room and outside of it, in venues such as the emergency department (ED), the critical care units, and the hospital wards. These distinctions were briefly mentioned in Chapter 8, and are summarized in Table 9.2. Airway management in these nonsurgical settings tends to be emergent, or at least urgent, depriving the physician of the time necessary to evaluate the patient fully and plan his or her intervention. Furthermore, each patient is presumed to have a full stomach during emergency airway management, and therefore must undergo rapid sequence intubation, with its attendant time pressure and requirement for cricoid pressure, which may distort the view of the glottis. Outside of the OR, intubation is usually carried out on the basis of patient need, whether for airway patency and protection or acute respiratory failure, whereas in the OR, patients are usually intubated to guarantee airway protection and ventilation during a reversible, pharmacologically-maintained anesthetic state. This leads to a strong emphasis, in the ASA algorithm, on preserving the option of re-emergence from anesthesia if intubation difficulty is encountered (Fig. 9.1) (3). This approach is impractical in the emergency department, or acute airway management elsewhere in the hospital, because the patient's pathology usually dictates that a definitive airway be rapidly obtained by whatever means possible. Finally, the orientation towards the emergent surgical airway is different among anesthesiologists and emergency physicians, as the latter generally have more training in cricothyrotomy.

Algorithms also exist to assist in decision making for airway management by emergency physicians. Walls, in his text on airway management in the ED, recommends the use of a "Universal Algorithm" for deciding the best means of managing a patient under emergent circumstances, along with several more specific algorithms for consideration in a variety of circumstances, such as an anticipated difficult airway, and the failure to secure the airway by direct laryngoscopy (Fig. 9.2) (6). These guidelines appear to represent a more realistic application of principles and constraints that pertain to physicians in the emergency setting.

AMERICAN SOCIETY OF ANESTHESIOLOGISTS

DIFFICULT AIRWAY ALGORITHM

1. Assess the likelihood and clinical impact of basic management problems:
   A. Difficult Ventilation
   B. Difficult Intubation
   C. Difficulty with Patient Cooperation or Consent
   D. Difficult Tracheostomy

2. Actively pursue opportunities to deliver supplemental oxygen throughout the process of difficult airway management

3. Consider the relative merits and feasibility of basic management choices:

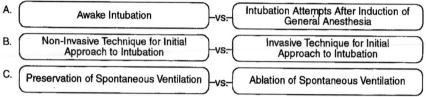

4. Develop primary and alternative strategies:

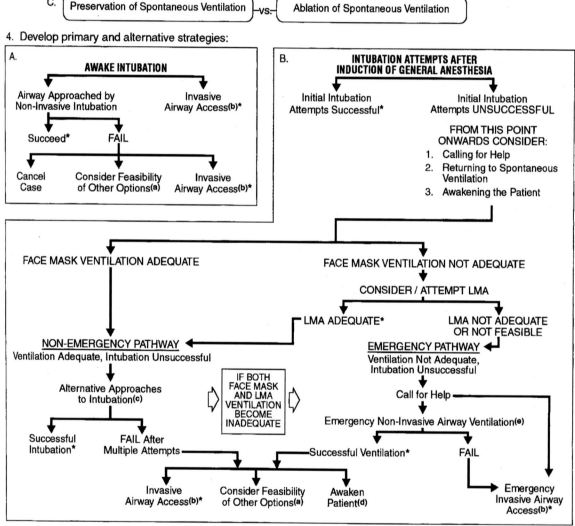

Figure 9.1 American Society of Anesthesiology difficult airway management algorithm. (From Practice guidelines for management of the difficult airway: an updated report by the ASA task force on management of the difficult airway. *Anesthesiology* 2003;98:1269–1277, with permission.)

Table 9.2

Differences in Airway Management Requirements Between Elective OR Cases and Emergency Situations

Aspects of Airway Management	Elective Cases in OR	Emergent Cases
Goals	Assure patent airway and ventilation while patient is unconscious	Obtain definitive airway, ensure ongoing ventilation and oxygenation, control secretions
Patient Characteristics	Respiratory system intact	Respiratory failure common
	Fasted	Presumed full stomach
	Infrequent C-spine immobilization	C-spine immobilization common
Preparatory time	Hours to days	Seconds to minutes
Alternatives for failed airway	Emphasis on awakening patient to allow resumption of spontaneous ventilation	Must progress to definitive airway

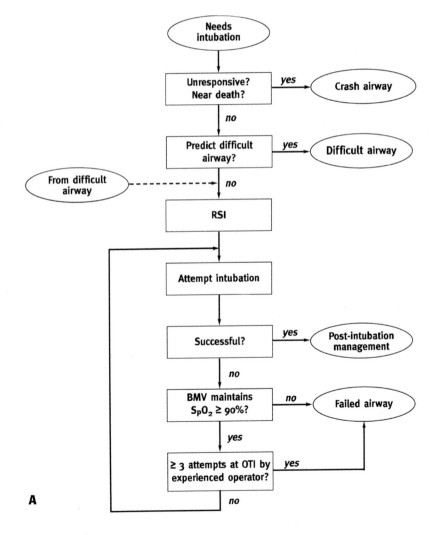

Figure 9.2 A–D. Emergency medicine airway management algorithms. (From Walls RM, ed. *Manual of airway management*, 2nd edition. Philadelphia: Lippincott Williams & Wilkins; 2004:8–21, with permission.)

Figure 9.2 (*continued*)

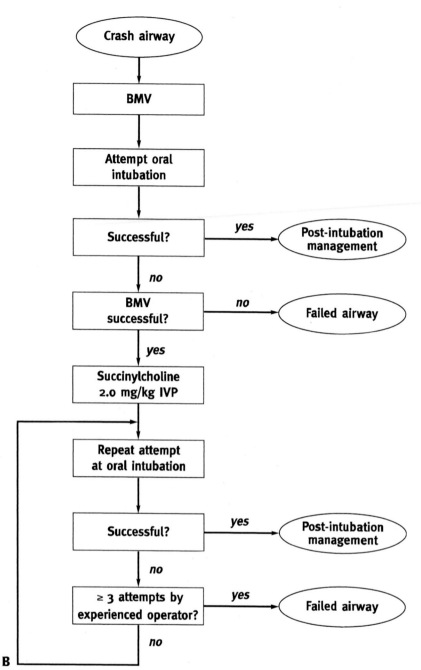

Figure 9.2 *(continued)*

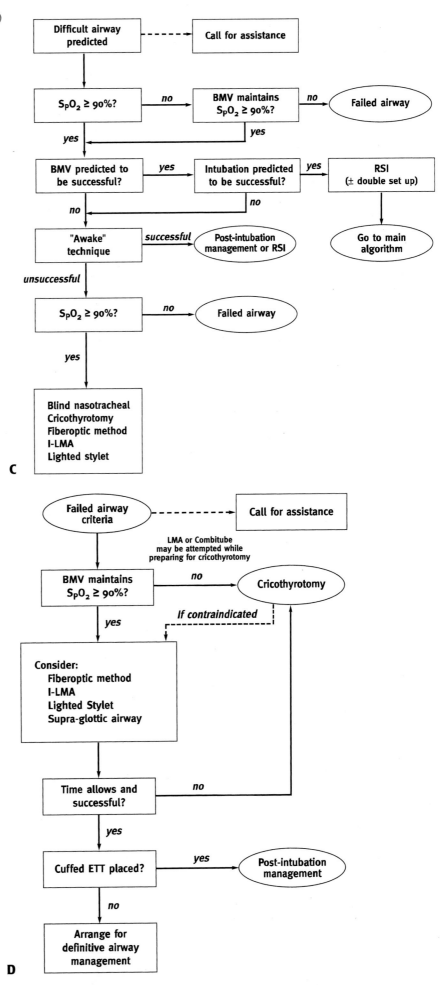

REFERENCES:

1. Benumof JL. Management of the difficult airway. *Anesthesiology* 1991;75;1087–1110.
2. Benumof JL, Dagg R, Benumof R. Critical hemoglobin desaturation will occur before return to an uparalyzed state following 1 mg/kg of intravenous succinylcholine. *Anesthesiology* 1997;87:979–982.
3. Caplan RA, Benumof JL, Berry FA, et al. Practice guidelines for management of the difficult airway: an updated report by the ASA task force on management of the difficult airway. *Anesthesiology* 2003;98:1269–1277.
4. Caplan RA, Benumof JL, Berry FA, et al. Practice guidelines for management of the difficult airway: a report by the ASA task force on management of the difficult airway. *Anesthesiology* 1993;78:597–602.
5. Peterson GN, Domino KB, Caplan RA, et al. Management of the difficult airway: a closed claims analysis. *Anesthesiology* 2005;103:33–39.
6. Walls RM. The emergency airway algorithms. In: Walls RM, ed. *Manual of airway management*, 2nd ed. Philadelphia: Lippincott William & Wilkins; 2004:8–21

Training in Airway Management

10

At the University of Pittsburgh Medical Center (UPMC), simulation plays an essential role in airway management training. At a newly-created simulation institute (WISER), students, residents, and fellows in a broad spectrum of health care professions and medical specialties undergo training in crisis management (1). Sim-man and Air-man simulators (Laerdahl Medical Corporation, Gatesville, TX) provide the means to instruct trainees in bag-mask ventilation, direct laryngoscopy, and difficult airway management (Fig. 10.1).

Medical students at our institution begin training in airway management during the second year, as part of a clinical procedures course. The first of five half-day training sessions focuses on bag-mask ventilation. These skills are accentuated and reinforced during the two-week, mandatory anesthesiology clerkship during the third year, which includes four operating room (OR)-based simulation sessions during which skills in both bag-mask ventilation and endotracheal tube (ETT) placement are stressed (2). Finally, in the fourth year anesthesiology elective, medical students again undergo four simulation sessions, one of which involves experience in advanced airway management, including the laryngeal mask airway, esophageal-tracheal combitube, intubating laryngeal mask airway, and trans-tracheal jet ventilation (Fig. 10.2).

For anesthesiology residents, airway management training is based upon the American Society of Anesthesiology difficult airway management algorithm (3). Trainees prepare for the course (two half-day sessions) with online didactic materials, and must pass a pre-test in order to participate. Each resident is faced with a series of scenarios, presented by a facilitator, simulating different arms of the algorithm. Thereafter, testing scenarios are presented, with each requiring specified critical actions for successful completion. Scenarios are pre-programmed into the simulator, ensuring consistency from one facilitator to the next.

Anesthesiology faculty undergo difficult airway management training in the simulation center as well. Schaefer et al have identified significant deficits in attending anesthesiologists' knowledge and application of the ASA difficult airway management algorithm during programmed simulations (4).

Emergency medicine residents at UPMC also undergo training with simulation to hone skills in airway management. An algorithm provides the framework for expected decision making patterns (5). Likewise, the department of critical care medicine has developed a guideline for airway management decisions that reflects the specific demands and patient characteristics of the intensive care arena. Residents in pediatrics and pediatric critical care fellows also undergo simulation-based difficult airway management instruction, utilizing the new Sim-baby simulator (Laerdal Medical Corporation, Gatesville, TX) (Fig.10.3) (6).

Anesthesiology residents additionally participate in focused sessions in fiberoptic bronchoscopic intubation (Fig. 10.4). The motor skills and eye-hand coordination necessary to accurately control the tip of the fiberscope require intense training and repeated practice sessions (7). Specific, repetitive drills requiring the operator to negotiate a series of obstacles, steering the fiberscope tip toward a target or series of targets, have proven effective in developing these skills. Video systems appear to facilitate skill acquisition in use of the fiberoptic bronchoscope for intubation (8).

Innovations that permit video imaging during direct laryngoscopy may eventually impact student and resident training in airway management. Recently, a new modality, termed video-laryngoscopy, has been developed that allows the instructor and the laryngoscopist-in-training to simultaneously visualize the pharynx and larynx during laryngoscopy. This has proven advantageous for instructing trainees and in directing the application of external laryngeal manipulation to provide the best view of the larynx during laryngoscopy (9). Examples of this type of device include the Video MacIntosh Laryngoscope system by Karl Storz Endoscopy (Tuttlingen, Germany) (Fig. 10.5) and the GlideScope (Saturn Biomedical, Burnaby, British Colombia, Canada).

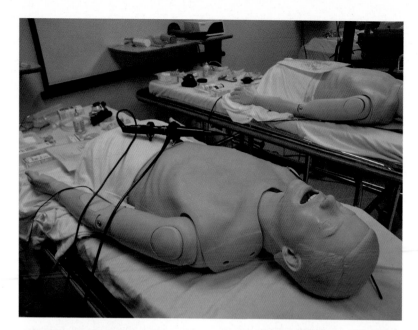

Figure 10.1 Air-man simulator (Laerdal Medical Corporation, Gatesville, TX).

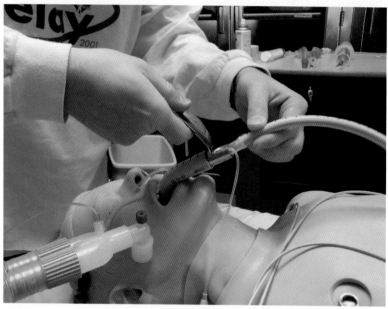

Figure 10.2 Difficult airway management training in the WISER center. A senior medical student learns to place an intubating LMA device.

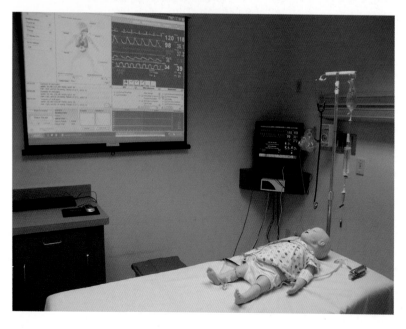

Figure 10.3 Sim-baby pediatric simulator (Laerdal Medical Corporation, Gatesville, TX).

Figure 10.4 Anesthesiology resident in the fiberoptic bronchoscopy intubation training course.

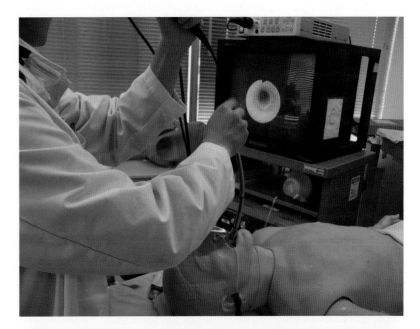

Figure 10.5 Karl Storz Endoscopy Video MacIntosh Intubation Laryngoscope System (Karl Storz Endoscopy, Tuttlingen, Germany). A camera is incorporated into the handle of the laryngoscope, which can be used in either MacIntosh 3 or 4 sizes. The laryngoscopic view is displayed on a monitor which can be at the bedside, allowing direction of a trainee, or placed overtop the patient during intubation, for better viewing by the laryngoscopist himself/herself.

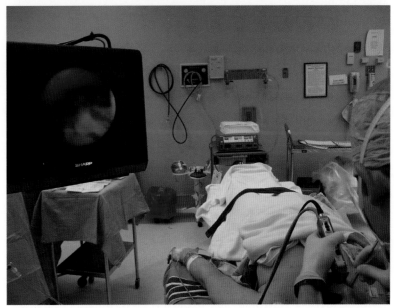

REFERENCES:

1. Schaefer JJ, Gonzales R. Dynamic simulation: a new tool for difficult airway training of professional health care providers. *Am J Anesth* 2000;27:232–242.
2. McIvor WR. Experience with medical student simulation education. *Crit Care Med* 2004;32:S66–69.
3. Practice guidelines for management of the difficult airway: an updated report by the ASA task force on management of the difficult airway. *Anesthesiology* 2003;98: 1269–1277.
4. Schaffer JJ. Mandatory competence-based difficult airway management training at the University of Pittsburgh department of anesthesiology-preliminary findings. Abstract presentation at International Meeting Medical Simulation, Albuquerque, NM, 2004.
5. Personal Communication. Paul Phrampus, MD, Director of WISER simulation center. February, 2006.
6. Fiodor ML. Pediatric simulation: a valuable tool for pediatric medical simulation. *Crit Care Med* 2004;32(S):S72–74.
7. Ovassapian A, Wheeler M. Fiberoptic endoscopy-aided techniques. In: Benumof JL, ed. *Airway management: principles and practice.* St. Louis: Mosby; 1996:282–319.
8. Wheeler M, Roth AG, Dsida RM, et al. Teaching residents pediatric fiberoptic intubation of the trachea. *Anesthesiology* 2004;101:842–846.
9. Kaplan MB, Ward DS, Berci G. A new video laryngoscope—an aid in intubation and teaching. *J Clin Anesth* 2002;14:620–626.

11

Examples and Illustrations of Conditions Predisposing to Difficult Airway Management

ANATOMIC ABNORMALITIES

Limited Mouth Opening

Limitations in mouth opening impede the ability of the laryngoscopist to visualize pharyngeal or laryngeal structures. Ideally, mouth opening should exceed 6 cm or 3 fingerbreadths (Fig. 11.1).

Disproportionally Large Tongue

Direct laryngoscopy requires that the tongue be forced into the floor of the mouth to permit the laryngoscopist to view the glottis. The larger the tongue, the more difficult this becomes, contributing to poor laryngoscopy grades. The disproportionally large tongue is usually evident when the Mallampati class is evaluated (Fig. 11.2).

Dental Abnormalities

Large, protruding teeth, or teeth lying at odd angles may complicate attempts to place the laryngoscope in the mouth, visualize the laryngeal orifice, or place the endotracheal tube (Figs. 11.3 and 11.4).

Abnormal Neck Size or Mobility

Patients with short, thick necks may present difficulty in achieving normal extension, and frequently have worse laryngoscopy grades at direct laryngoscopy than patients with long, thin necks (Fig. 11.5).

Mandibular Size

The small mandible, or receding chin, adversely affects the ability to visualize the glottis (Fig. 11.6).

Epiglottis

Occasionally, the elongated epiglottis is difficult to elevate with the curved blade, and a straight blade must be utilized to lift it directly out of the way (Fig. 11.7).

Nasal Turbinates

Prominent or protuberant nasal turbinates may create an obstruction to passage of nasopharyngeal airways or nasal endotracheal tubes (ETTs), leading to trauma with severe epistaxis (Fig. 11.8).

Facial Hair

Bushy beards or goatees may complicate attempts to make a seal with the face mask, resulting in difficult mask ventilation (Fig. 11.9).

CONGENITAL ANOMALIES

Many congenital anomalies affecting facial, oral, pharyngeal, or cervical structures create challenging intubating conditions.

Oral Cavity

Some congenital abnormalities result in enlargement of the tongue, as is commonly seen in Down's syndrome (Fig. 11.10).

Larynx

Airway stenosis may be a congenital condition (Fig. 11.11).

Cervical Spine

Cervical spine skeletal anomalies may complicate attempts to manage the airway by conventional means (Fig. 11.12).

Facial Skeleton

Abnormalities of the maxilla or mandible can complicate face mask ventilation and direct laryngoscopy (Fig. 11.13).

Neck

Large congenital malformations may compromise the airway, necessitating tracheostomy (Fig. 11.14).

PATHOLOGY

Many diseases of the head, neck, and chest can adversely affect direct laryngoscopy.

Figure 11.1 Limited mouth opening.

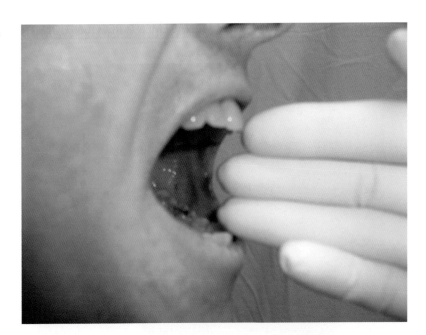

Figure 11.2 A disproportionally large tongue. (From Benjamin B, Bingham B, Hawke M, et al. *A color atlas of otorhino-laryngology*. Philadelphia: JB. Lippincott Co; 1995, with permission.)

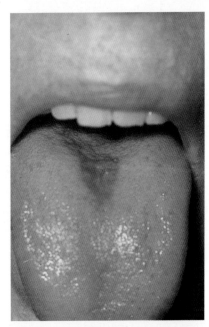

Figure 11.3 Large, protuberant incisor teeth.

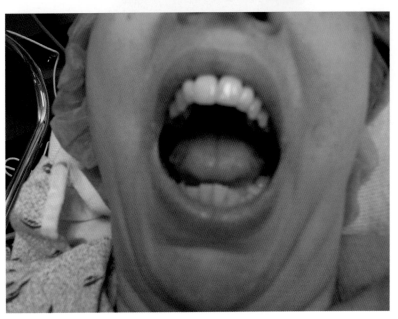

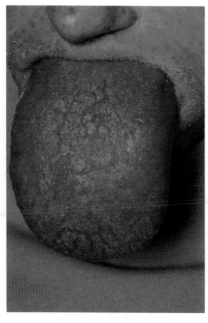

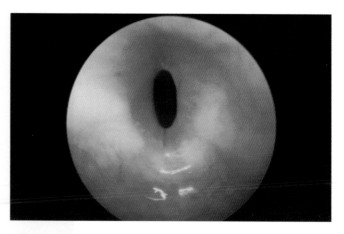

Figure 11.11 Congenital subglottic stenosis. (From Benjamin B, Bingham B, Hawke M, et al. *A color atlas of otorhinolaryngology*. Philadelphia: JB. Lippincott Co; 1995, with permission.)

Figure 11.10 Enlarged tongue in Down's syndrome. (From Benjamin B, Bingham B, Hawke M, et al. *A color atlas of otorhinolaryngology*. Philadelphia: JB. Lippincott Co; 1995, with permission.)

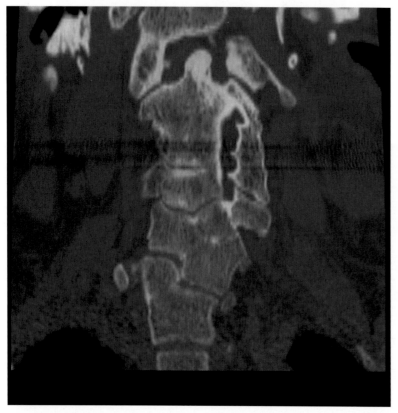

Figure 11.12 Severe cervical spine anomaly in Klippel-Feil syndrome. (Courtesy of Dr. Barton Branstetter, Department of Radiology, University of Pittsburgh Medical Center.)

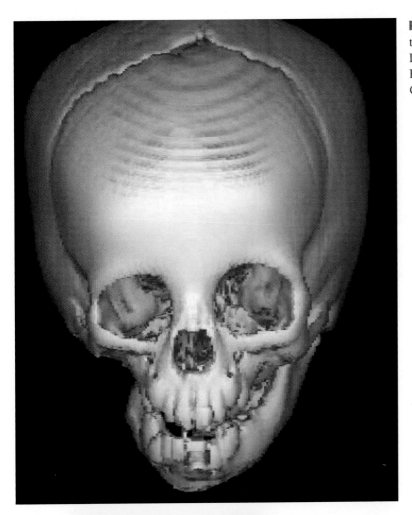

Figure 11.13 Congenital facial malformation evident on 3D CT scan. (Courtesy of Dr. Barton Branstetter, Department of Radiology, University of Pittsburgh Medical Center.)

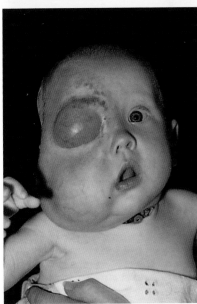

Figure 11.14 Congenital subglottic hemangioma which mandated tracheostomy in this infant. (From Benjamin B, Bingham B, Hawke M, et al. *A color atlas of otorhinolaryngology*. Philadelphia: JB. Lippincott Co; 1995, with permission.)

INFECTION

Epiglottitis

Infection of the epiglottis and supraglottic region can create life-threatening airway obstruction.

In epiglottitis, severe supraglottic edema and erythema may lead to airway obstruction, mandating endotracheal intubation by direct laryngoscopy, if possible, or by surgical means (Fig. 11.15A). A lateral soft tissue cervical radiograph usually reveals the "thumb sign" of an enlarged, inflamed epiglottis (Fig. 11.15B).

Ludwig's Angina

Infection of the floor of the mouth, usually an extension of dental infection ("trench mouth"), can cause severe pain on swallowing, trismus, and difficulty opening the mouth and displacing the tongue during direct laryngoscopy. Figure 11.16A shows a patient with swelling and erythema of the submandibular space, a manifestation of Ludwig's angina. Figure 11.16B shows a computed tomography (CT) of a patient with Ludwig's angina. Note the extent of swelling and potential airway compromise.

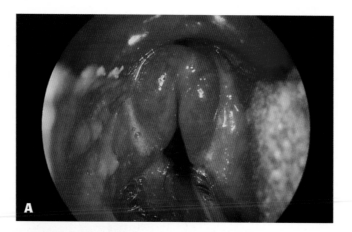

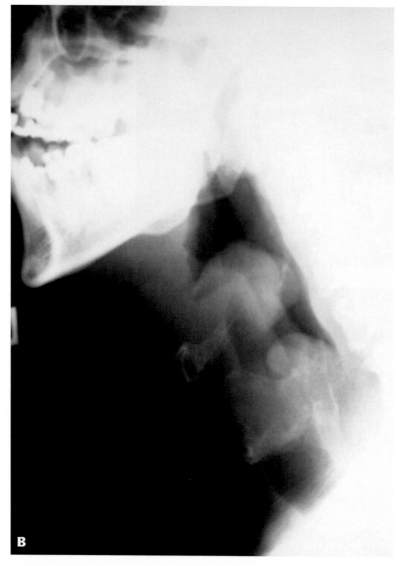

Figure 11.15 A. Severe supraglottic edema and erythema in acute epiglottitis. (From Benjamin B, Bingham B, Hawke M, et al. *A color atlas of otorhinolaryngology*. Philadelphia: JB. Lippincott Co; 1995, with permission.) B. Enlarged, "thumb-shaped" epiglottis evident on lateral soft-tissue cervical radiograph. (Courtesy of Dr. Barton Branstetter, Department of Radiology, University of Pittsburgh Medical Center.)

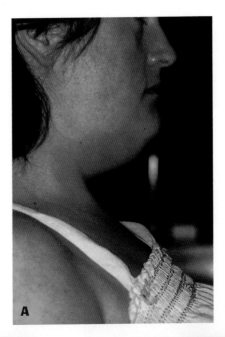

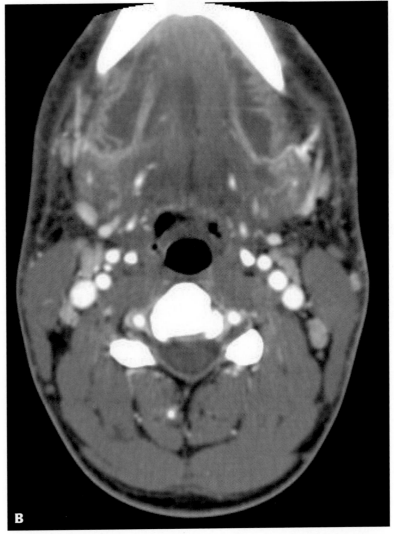

Figure 11.16 **A.** Swelling and erythema of the submandibular space. (From Benjamin B, Bingham B, Hawke M, et al. *A color atlas of otorhinolaryngology.* Philadelphia: JB. Lippincott Co; 1995, with permission). **B.** CT of a patient with Ludwig's angina. (Courtesy of Dr. Barton Branstetter, Department of Radiology, University of Pittsburgh Medical Center.)

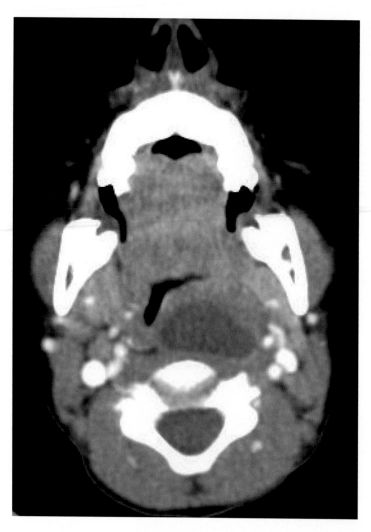

Figure 11.17 Retropharyngeal abscess. (Courtesy of Dr. Barton Branstetter, Department of Radiology, University of Pittsburgh Medical Center.)

Retropharyngeal Abscess

This process, most common in young children, causes neck stiffness and bulging of the posterior pharyngeal wall. In Figure 11.17, a CT of a patient with retropharyngeal abscess shows marked prevertebral edema and narrowing of the upper airway.

Dental Abscess

Large abscesses may lead to trismus and distortion of intra-oral structures. Figure 11.18 shows a patient with a dental abscess who has significant jaw swelling and is likely to have trismus.

Peritonsillar Abscess

An abscess in the tonsillar fossa often results in drooling, trismus, odynophagia, and bulging of the soft palate of the affected side. Figure 11.19 depicts a peritonsillar abscess with bulging soft palate and copious exudate.

NEOPLASMS

Supraglottic Cancer

Carcinoma of the pre-epiglottic space, shown in Figure 11.20, makes direct laryngoscopy difficult, particularly with a curved blade.

Laryngeal Carcinoma

Carcinomas of the larynx may be relatively silent until they have progressed to significant airway obstruction (Fig. 11.21).

Nasopharyngeal Carcinoma

Like other airway tumors, nasopharyngeal carcinoma may become extensive before discovery. In this magnetic resonance image (MRI), widespread involvement of the nasopharynx is evident (Fig. 11.22).

Figure 11.18 Dental abscess with significant jaw swelling. (From Benjamin B, Bingham B, Hawke M, et al. *A color atlas of otorhinolaryngology*. Philadelphia: JB. Lippincott Co; 1995, with permission.)

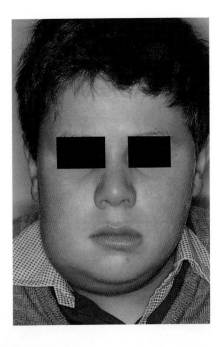

Figure 11.19 Peritonsillar abscess.

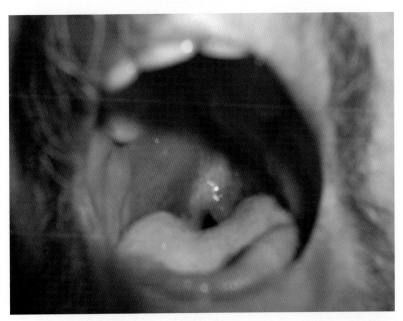

Figure 11.20 Carcinoma of the pre-epiglottic space. (From Benjamin B, Bingham B, Hawke M, et al. *A color atlas of otorhinolaryngology*. Philadelphia: JB. Lippincott Co; 1995, with permission.)

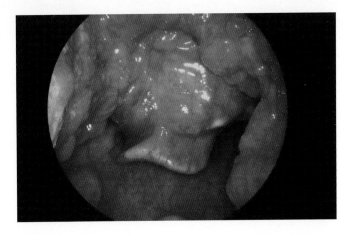

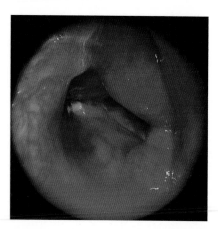

Figure 11.21 Laryngeal carcinoma. (From Benjamin B, Bingham B, Hawke M, et al. *A color atlas of otorhinolaryngology.* Philadelphia; JB. Lippincott Co; 1995, with permission.)

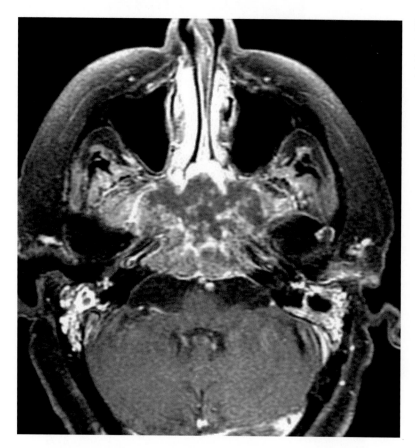

Figure 11.22 Nasopharyngeal carcinoma. (Courtesy of Dr. Barton Branstetter, Department of Radiology, University of Pittsburgh Medical Center.)

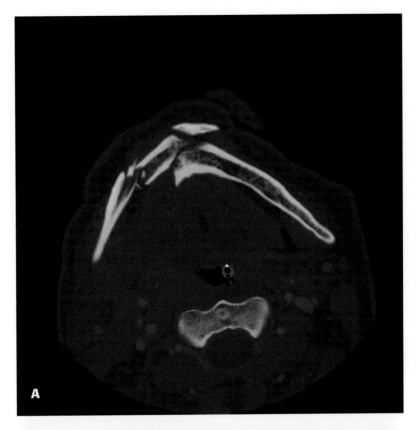

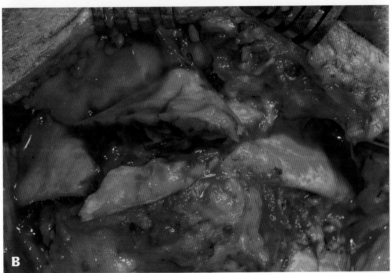

Figure 11.23 A. Severely comminuted mandibular fracture. B. Surgical repair of fracture pictured in Figure 11.23A. (Courtesy of Lison Yeung, DDS and Dr. William Chung, Department of Oromaxillofacial Surgery, University of Pittsburgh School of Medicine.)

TRAUMA

Mandibular Fracture

Mandibular fracture usually results in trismus, edema, and distortion of intra-oral structures. This may make direct laryngoscopy and intubation by the oral route difficult. Figure 11.23A shows a CT scan of a severe, comminuted

mandibular fracture. The supporting ring of the mandible is lost, resulting in a "flail mandible." Figure 11.23B depicts the surgical repair of the comminuted fracture shown in Figure 11.23A.

Facial Fractures

Bleeding, edema, loss of anatomic landmarks, and airway obstruction combine to make management of the airway very challenging in these patients. If the airway is inacces-

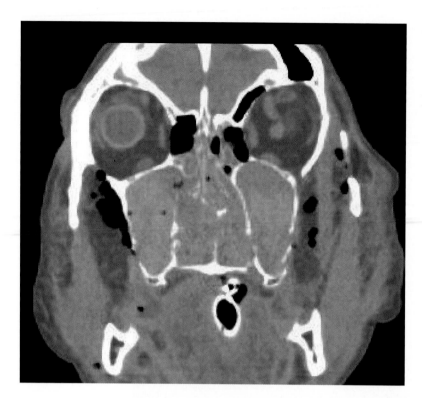

Figure 11.24 A LeFort I fracture of the midface. Multiple nasal fractures and maxillary sinuses filled with blood are evident on this coronal CT scan. (Courtesy of Dr. Barton Branstetter, Department of Radiology, University of Pittsburgh Medical Center.)

sible or unrecognizable, surgical airway is necessary (Fig. 11.24).

Cervical Spine Fracture/Dislocation

Recognized or potential cervical spine injury mandates extreme care with airway management. Cervical spine flexion or extension may result in spinal cord injury. In-line cervical immobilization is typically utilized in the trauma patient with potential spine injury who requires intubation for airway control. Patients with known cervical spine injury are managed with fiberoptic flexible or rigid optical scopes, or other forms of intubation that re-

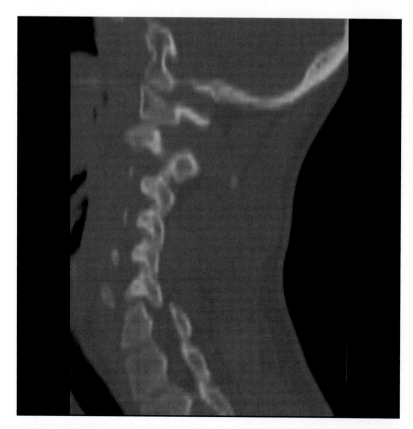

Figure 11.25 This tomogram shows marked anterior displacement of C6 on C7 due to bilateral facet dislocation. (Courtesy of Dr. Barton Branstetter, Department of Radiology, University of Pittsburgh Medical Center.)

quire no significant motion of the cervical spine (Fig. 11.25).

Laryngeal Injury

Blunt injury to the larynx may result in fractures of the cartilages or disruption of the airway. Airway management attempts with direct laryngoscopy may fail or worsen the injury. Figure 11.26 shows a laryngeal fracture. Disruption of the laryngeal cartilages is evident in this CT of the larynx. Tracheostomy may be necessary in such patients, until surgical repair can be undertaken.

EDEMA

Edema of the oral cavity, neck, larynx, or pharynx from a variety of causes may compromise the airway and complicate attempts at face mask ventilation and direct laryngoscopy (Figs. 11.27 to 11.29).

ARTHRITIS/BONEY HYPERTROPHY

Arthritic changes of the temporomandibular joints, the atlanto-occipital joint, or the joints of the cervical spine can make direct laryngoscopy very challenging and may mandate awake intubation, depending on the degree of instability or restriction of motion (Figs. 11.30 and 11.31).

MISCELLANEOUS

Hematoma, tissue infiltration, or hypertrophy of tissues involving the airway may distort structures, restrict range of motion, or reduce the space available for viewing or placement of airway management tools (Figs. 11.32 to 11.34).

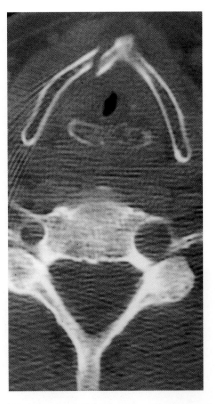

Figure 11.26 Laryngeal fracture. (From Benjamin B, Bingham B, Hawke M, et al. *A color atlas of otorhinolaryngology*. Philadelphia: JB. Lippincott Co; 1995, with permission.)

Figure 11.27 Postoperative neck edema from shoulder arthroscopy. This can become severe enough to shift the trachea and occlude the airway.

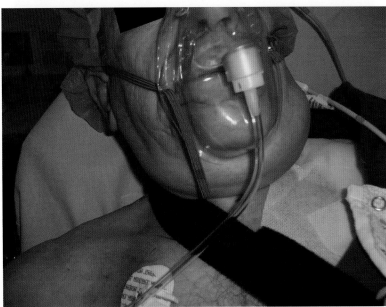

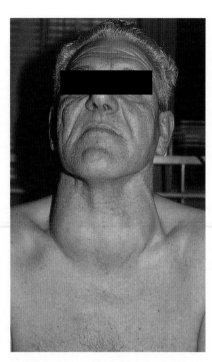

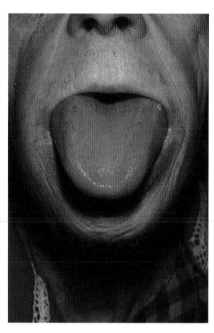

Figure 11.33 Markedly enlarged thyroid gland. (From Benjamin B, Bingham B, Hawke M, et al. *A color atlas of otorhinolaryngology*. Philadelphia: JB. Lippincott Co; 1995, with permission.)

Figure 11.34 Enlargement of the tongue in amyloidosis. (From Benjamin B, Bingham B, Hawke M, et al. *A color atlas of otorhinolaryngology*. Philadelphia: JB. Lippincott Co; 1995, with permission.)

Mirrors and Mirror Blades

Concept: Mirrors have been used to facilitate endotracheal tube (ETT) placement when the glottis is difficult to visualize. These include blades with an integral mirror that provide an inverted view of the glottis, such as the Siker Blade (1) (Fig. 12.1). The Neustein Blade involves a mirrored attachment to the MacIntosh blade that includes a guide channel for a stylet, over which the ETT is passed after the blade is removed (2). Both of these devices result in the laryngoscopist viewing an inverted image, making their initial use cumbersome. Neither is frequently used in clinical practice.

Evidence: The evidence for the use of mirror blades is anecdotal, rather than comparative. Siker, in his original description of the blade, described 99% success in intubating a series of 100 patients, including several cases in which standard blades had provided a poor view of the larynx (1).

Preparation for Direct Laryngoscopy with Siker Blade:

Standard preparations for direct laryngoscopy (Chapter 3)
Place the mirror blade for several minutes in warm water before use, to avoid fogging, or apply defogging solution.

Procedure to Attempt Direct Laryngoscopy (Figs. 12.2 and 12.3):

Establish inadequate view of larynx
Attach Siker blade to laryngoscope handle

Perform direct laryngoscopy
Note inverted image of larynx in mirror of blade
Place endotracheal tube using mirror for visualization
Inflate cuff, confirm ETT placement
Fix ETT in place

Practicality: Portable, affordable
Relatively simple conceptually
Unfamiliar due to inverted image, requires practice

Indications: Poor laryngoscopy grade

Contraindications: Usual contraindications to direct laryngoscopy (Chapter 3)
Lack of familiarity with device
Inaccessibility of oral cavity

Complications: Similar to those of direct laryngoscopy (Chapter 3)
Inability to place endotracheal tube using inverted image
Fogging of mirror, obscuring image

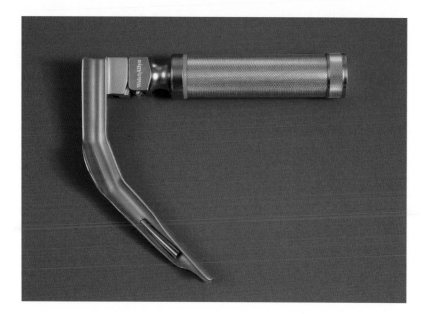

Figure 12.1 The Siker blade.

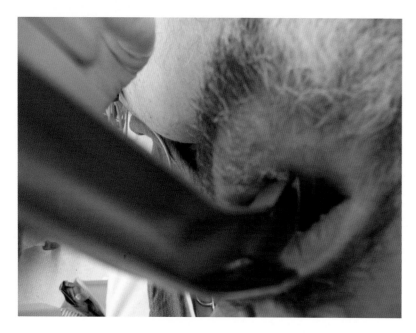

Figure 12.2 Insertion of the Siker blade into the mouth. Note the relatively high vertical profile of the blade.

Figure 12.3 Grade 2 view of the glottis as reflected in the mirror of the Siker blade.

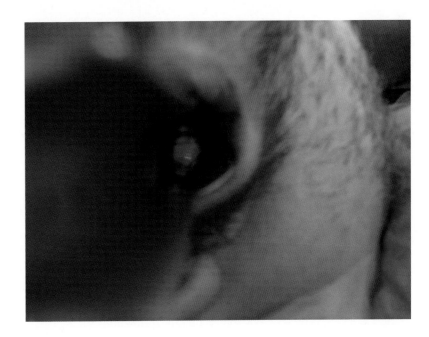

REFERENCES:

1. Siker ES. A mirror laryngoscope. *Anesthesiology* 1956; 17:38–42.

2. Neustein SM. The Neustein laryngoscope: A new solution to the difficult intubation. *Anesth Rev* 1992;19:54–59.

13

Prisms and Prism Blades

Concept: Initial use of the optical prism for airway visualization dates to the early 20th century, but little development of the technique occurred until the late 1960s when Huffman described a prism made from Plexiglass for attachment to the standard MacIntosh blade, which provides 30 degrees of light refraction (1). This helps the laryngoscopist gain a view of the glottic opening when a grade 3 or 4 view is present, possibly facilitating intubation (Figs. 13.1 to 13.4). These prisms are readily available today, at low cost, but fogging can be troublesome unless the prism is warmed before use, or a defogging solution is applied to prevent this. The prisms may reduce the room needed for manipulation of the endotracheal tube (ETT) in the mouth.

Of recent interest is a blade specifically designed to incorporate a prism if the view is unsatisfactory during direct laryngoscopy. Deemed the Belscope, it is a straight blade with a 45-degree angulation at its midpoint, and is available in three sizes (2) (Fig. 13.5). The blade's effectiveness has been evaluated by its originator, for whom it is named, and has been applied successfully in patients with normal anatomy as well as those with difficult airways (3).

Evidence: No comparative trials of prisms are available. Efficacy of these devices has been established only anecdotally. In his original description of the device, Huffman reported he was able to effectively visualize the glottic opening with the prism device in each of 35 patients, including those with large, protuberant teeth (1). Bellhouse reported his experience with more than 3,500 intubations using his blade, and reported it "wholly successful." In 12 cases of failure of the MacIntosh blade, and 7 cases of known or encountered difficulty with direct laryngoscopy, the blade was effective (2). Only rarely was the prism used.

Preparation (Figs. 13.1 and 13.2):

Standard preparations for direct laryngoscopy (see Chapter 3)
If a prism is to be used, it should be heated, or a defogging solution applied

Procedure (Figs. 13.3 and 13.4):

Conduct direct laryngscopy, establish poor view
Place prism on vertical flange of MacIntosh blade
Repeat laryngoscopy, using view through prism to bring glottis into view
Visualize ETT placement through prism
Inflate tube cuff, ventilate and confirm ETT placement

Practicality: Inexpensive
Simple in concept
Portable; but small prisms are frequently misplaced
Not familiar; requires practice in vivo and in vitro

Indications: Poor laryngoscopic view (grade 3 or 4 view)

Contraindications: Similar to those of direct laryngoscopy (see Chapter 3)
Lack of familiarity with device
Inaccessibility of oral cavity

Complications: Same as for direct laryngoscopy (see Chapter 3)
Fogging of prism, obscuring view
Inability to place ETT, due to unfamiliar viewing characteristics

Figure 13.1 Prism for 3 MacIntosh blade.

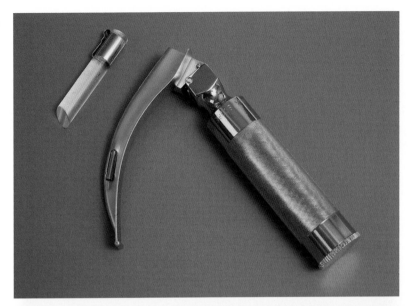

Figure 13.2 Prism for 3 MacIntosh blade, mounted.

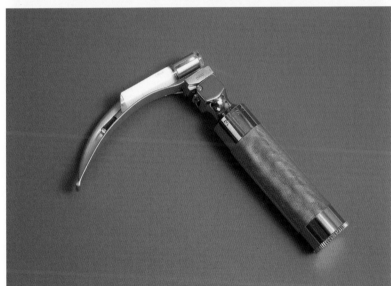

Figure 13.3 Laryngoscopy with prism on 3 MacIntosh blade, showing view through prism: the airway is evident as grade 2 view.

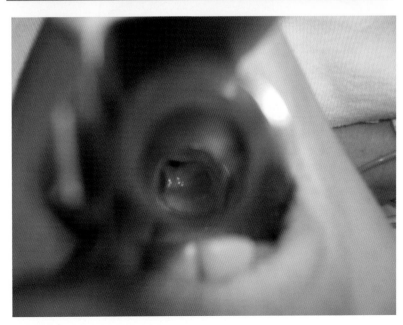

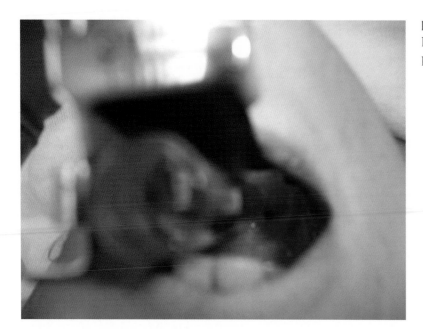

Figure 13.4 The vantage point of the laryngoscopist, without looking through the prism: a poor view of the larynx is evident.

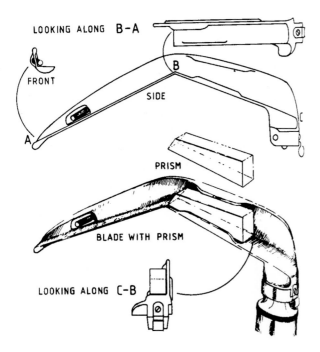

Figure 13.5 Diagram of Bellscope laryngoscope blade with prism in place. (From Bellhouse CP. An angulated laryngoscope for routine and difficult tracheal intubation. *Anesthesiology* 1988;69:126–129, with permission.)

REFERENCES:

1. Huffman JP. The application of prisms to curved laryngoscopes. *J Am Assoc Nurse Anesth* 1968;36:138–139.
2. Bellhouse CP. An angulated laryngoscope for routine and difficult tracheal intubation. *Anesthesiology* 1988;69:126–129.
3. Mayall RM. The Belscope for management of the difficult airway. *Anesthesiology* 1992;76:1059–1060.

14

Bougies and Airway Stylets

Concept: At times it is beneficial to insert a guiding catheter, or introducer (sometimes referred to as a "bougie") (Fig. 14.1), into the glottis before inserting the endotracheal tube (ETT) by sliding it over the stylet. These devices provide a means to intubate during direct laryngoscopy when the glottic opening is not well visualized, but its location is inferred from the view of the interarytenoid notch or the epiglottis (a grade 3 or 4 laryngoscopic view). The malleable Eschmann introducer, with its stiff, angulated distal tip, lends itself to this task because it is small enough to be maneuvered in the pharynx, where it is used to "probe" for the glottic opening, and its end is firm enough to rattle against the tracheal rings as it is placed in the airway, providing a sense of correct placement. It is frequently used in the UK for difficult airway management. The Frova intubating stylet (Cook Critical Care, Bloomington, IN) similarly facilitates intubation when the glottic view is poor. This device is a hollow cannula with a malleable, removable steel stylet, which permits "jet" (high pressure) ventilation through an adaptor, or oxygen insufflation during intubation attempts. Airway exchange catheters can also be used as ETT introducers. These permit attachment to an anesthetic circuit, resuscitation bag, or high-pressure ventilation system for ongoing ventilation if ETT insertion proves difficult or impossible after the introducer is inserted.

Evidence: Numerous case reports and case series attest to the value of the bougie or Eschmann stylet in difficult intubation in the operating room (OR), and more recently in emergency medicine practice (1–3). A few comparative studies have appeared. Nolan et al simulated cervical spine injury with in-line immobilization in 157 elective general anesthesia patients, and reported 100% success in intubation (during direct laryngoscopy) of 79 cases with the bougie, but only 93% success in 78 cases with an ETT, without use of the bougie (4). In another study of simulated difficult intubation, the authors reported success rates in intubation of only 66% with a styletted ETT, versus 96% with the bougie (5). Moscati reported the efficacy of this device in three cases in the emergency department (ED) in which the glottic inlet could not be visualized and intubation by direct laryngoscopy had repeatedly failed (6).

Preparation for Direct Laryngoscopy (Chapter 3):

Lubricate bougie lightly
Enlist aid of an assistant

Procedure (Figs. 14.2 to 14.8):

Proceed with direct laryngoscopy, establish poor view
Identify interarytenoid notch at back of glottis, if possible
Place distal (angulated) tip of bougie above notch, or below the epiglottis, if it is obstructing the view
Probe for opening of glottis
Gently insert bougie, feeling for tip against tracheal rings
If tip does not encounter rings, continue insertion
At approximately 28 cm to 30 cm, bougie will encounter resistance as it enters one of the bronchi and its tip encounters the smaller airways (this does not occur if bougie is placed in esophagus)
Pull bougie back from resistance
Have assistant place ETT over the proximal end of bougie
Assistant then holds proximal end of bougie, preventing its advance, as ETT is moved along it towards glottis
Leave laryngoscope in place, elevating soft tissues during advancement of the ETT
Guide ETT into glottis, maintaining position of bougie
Insert ETT to desired depth
Pull bougie back, remove from ETT
Inflate ETT cuff, confirm placement

Practicality: Simple concept, requires little practice
Relatively familiar
Portable
Readily affordable (typical Eschmann stylet is $40 to $60)

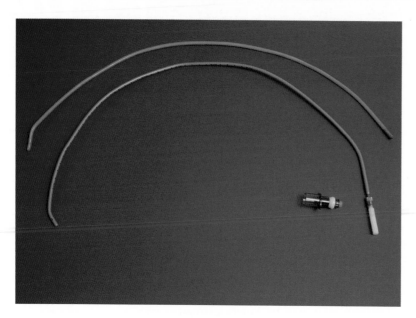

Figure 14.1 Eschmann stylet (*top*) and Frova intubating stylet (*bottom*) with attached adaptor for high-pressure oxygen insufflation, and 15 mm adaptor for attachment to anesthesia circuit or resuscitation bag (at bottom of photo).

Indications: Poor laryngoscopy grade during direct laryngoscopy

Suspected cervical spine injury, in a patient requiring intubation

Contraindications: Similar to those of direct laryngoscopy (see Chapter 3)

Laryngeal disruption

Inaccessibility of oral cavity

Complications: Misplacement of ETT into esophagus can occur

Tracheal rings may not be felt, even when placed correctly

Trauma to larynx or bronchus may occur

ETT can be advanced too far, into mainstem bronchus

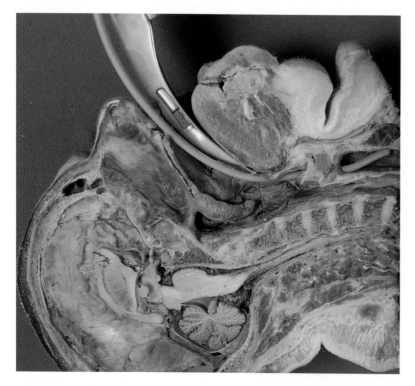

Figure 14.2 Direct laryngoscopy with insertion of bougie in a cadaver specimen.

Figure 14.3 Bougie placed into esophagus (no resistance would be met in this situation as the bougie is advanced).

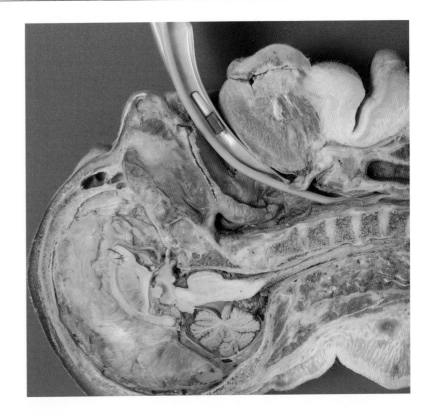

Figure 14.4 Sliding ETT over bougie.

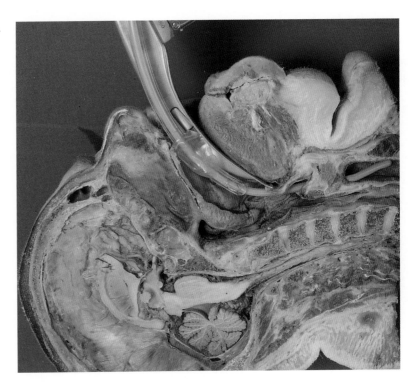

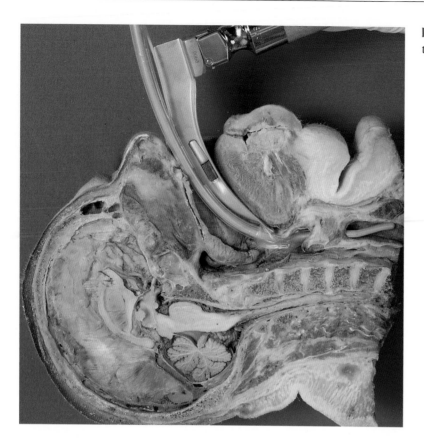

Figure 14.5 Passing ETT over bougie through the glottis.

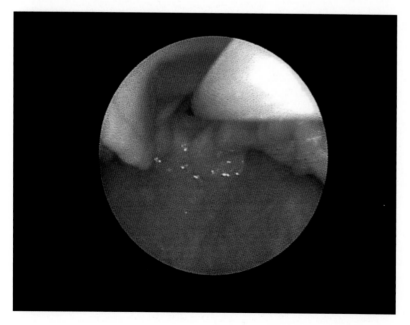

Figure 14.6 Placement of bougie into glottis during direct laryngoscopy.

Figure 14.7 Placing ETT over bougie with the help of an assistant.

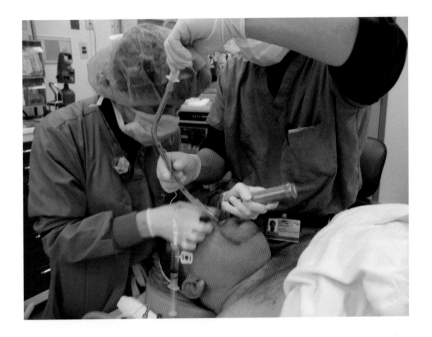

Figure 14.8 Sliding ETT into larynx over bougie (laryngoscope still in place to facilitate ETT entry into larynx).

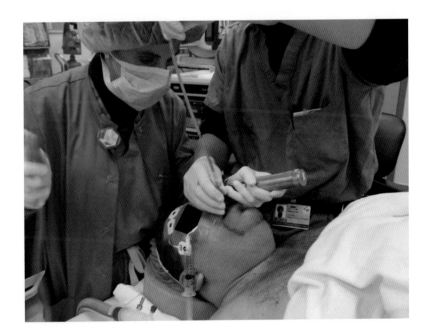

REFERENCES:

1. McCarroll SM, Lamont BJ, Buckland MR, et al. The gum elastic bougie: lod but still useful. *Anesthesiology* 1988;68: 643–644.
2. Nocera A. A flexible solution for emergency intubation difficulties. *Ann Emerg Med* 1996;27:665–677.
3. Dogra S, Faconer R, Latto IP. Successful difficult intubation. *Anaesthesia* 1990;45:774–776.
4. Nolan JP, Wilson ME. Orotracheal intubation in patients with potential cervical spine injury. *Anaesthesia* 1993;48: 630–633.
5. Gataure PS, Vaughan RS, Latto IP. Simulated difficult intubation: Comparison of the gum elastic bougie and the stylet. *Anaesthesia* 1996;51:935–938.
6. Moscati R, Jehle D, Christiansen G, et al. Endotracheal tube introducer for failed intubations: a variant of the gum elastic bougie. *Ann Emerg Med* 2000;36:52–56.

Blind Nasotracheal Intubation

Concept: Blind Nasotracheal Intubation (BNTI) remains a viable technique in the elective surgical patient and in emergency intubation, particularly for patients with challenging anatomy. In this procedure, an endotracheal tube (ETT) is placed through one of the nares into the nasopharynx (Fig. 15.1), then into the glottis, guided primarily by breath sounds, without visualization. At its best, it is a smooth, effective, and painless procedure. At its worst, BNTI is traumatic and uncomfortable, and may make subsequent attempts at airway management more difficult by causing epistaxis or vomiting. BNTI requires preservation of spontaneous ventilation, so that audible inspiratory efforts can be detected and synchronized with tube placement. It is much less likely to be successful in the apneic patient. The breath sounds, when optimized, help to guide the tube into a position just above the glottis, so that controlled advancement of the tube allows correct placement. Whistles are available to attach to the end of the ETT to make ventilation through the ETT more audible, confirming placement of the tube in the airway. BNTI is less likely to be used in children than in adults, due to the lack of cooperation, the small size of the nares, and frequent hypertrophy of the adenoidal tonsils.

Evidence: BNTI is supported anecdotally by case reports and case studies in both the emergency medicine and anesthesiology literature. In the National Emergency Airway Registry, this method was utilized in about 5% of all intubations, with a success rate of nearly 86% (1). In Dronen's comparison of BNTI to direct laryngoscopy for intubations in the emergency department (ED), the 68% rate of successful endotracheal intubation was significantly lower than that for direct laryngoscopy, in which there were no failures (2). In addition, complication rates, mostly nasal bleeding and emesis, were much higher with BNTI. When paramedics utilized BNTI in 219 intubations, the rate of appropriate ETT placement improved from 58% to 72% when a directional tip control tube was utilized (3). BNTI in children is typically reserved for cases in which other methods of intubation are not feasible (4).

Preparation (Figs. 15.2 and 15.3):

Soften the ETT in a warmed saline solution, if time

allows (directional ETTs tend to be very soft and do not require this step)

Check the patency of each nostril, through inquiry and physical exam (occluding each side and asking patient to breathe through the nose can be revealing)

Prepare the nose with local anesthetic gel or solution, and a vasoconstrictor (phenylephrine solution or oxymetazoline nasal spray)

Placement of successively larger nasopharyngeal airways, coated with local anesthetic and vasoconstrictor, reduces epistaxis in the elective situation.

Sedation or anesthesia may be provided, but spontaneous respiration should be preserved

Patient may be supine, or in seated position

Standard preparations should be made for direct laryngoscopy (see Chapter 3)

Procedure (Figs.15.4 to 15.8):

Place ETT in nares (the right nostril is usually chosen, to allow the bevel of ETT to approach the turbinates atraumatically)

The tube is directed along the floor of the nasal cavity, parallel to the hard palate

Place an ear near the proximal end of the ETT, listening carefully for breath sounds

When the nasopharynx is reached, breath sounds become audible

Gentle advancement of the tube should allow an increase in the sounds, as the glottis is approached

If breath sounds diminish, suspect the tube is advancing into the esophagus; withdraw and redirect or change head and neck position

When the breath sounds are maximal, the ETT is held in place

During the pause, breath sounds are carefully tracked

The tube should then be advanced as inspiration is initiated

If successful, patients breathe through the tube, and cannot phonate

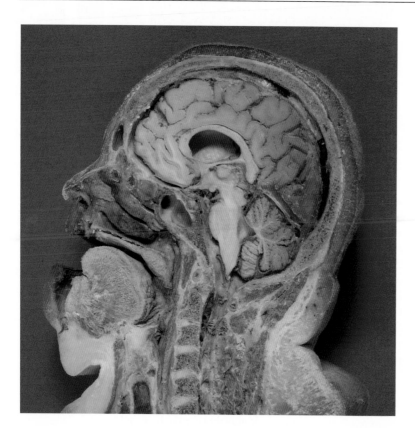

Figure 15.1 Sagittal section through cadaver specimen, showing floor of nasal cavity, turbinates, and nasopharynx: the path traveled by a nasotracheal tube.

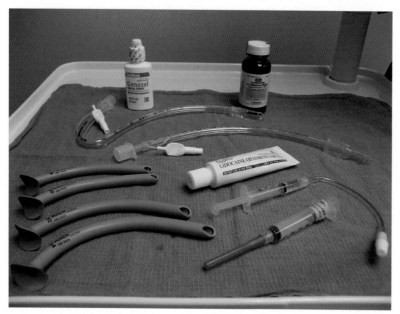

Figure 15.2 Preparation for BNTI: nasal airways, local anesthetic gel, and topical vasoconstrictor solutions.

Figure 15.3 Dilation of the nose with nasal airways/lubricants/vasoconstricors.

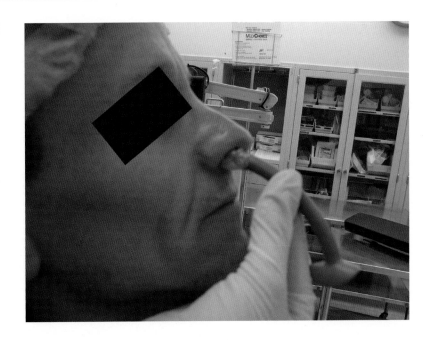

Figure 15.4 ETT insertion, along floor of nose.

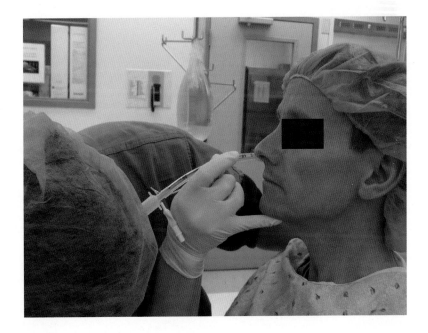

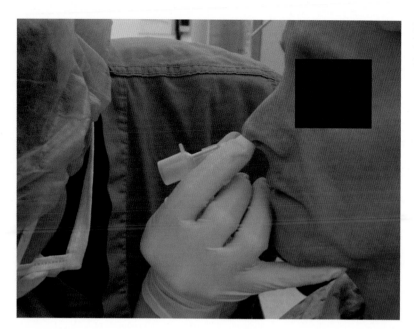

Figure 15.5 ETT in position in the hypopharynx: breath sounds should be maximally audible.

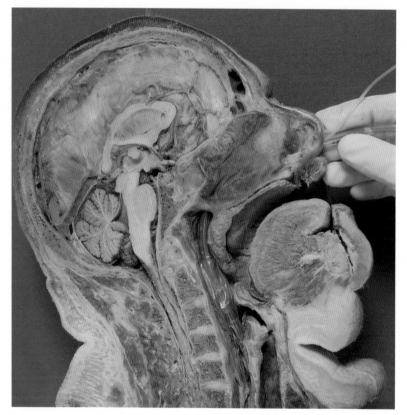

Figure 15.6 Tube misdirection (too far posterior). Neck extension will help to align the tube with the glottis.

Figure 15.7 Tube misdirection (too far anterior). In this setting, the tube may be palpable above the thyroid cartilage. Neck flexion will help to align the tube with the glottis.

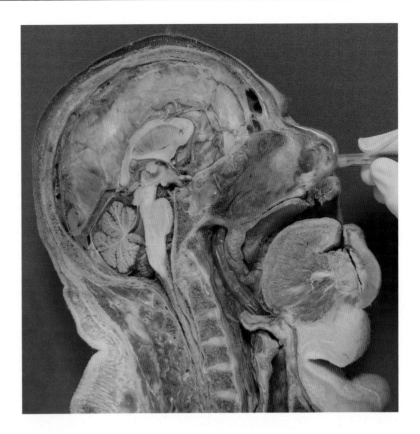

Figure 15.8 Correct position, advancing ETT into glottis.

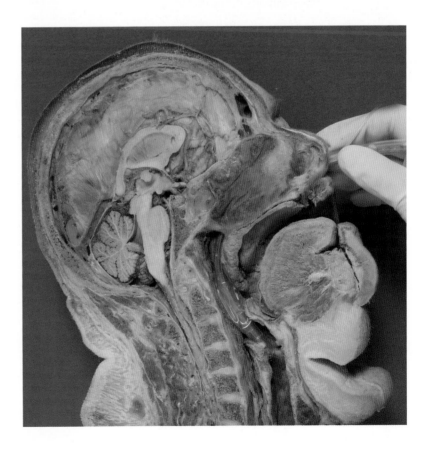

When unsuccessful, changes in head position may assist in correct tube placement: extension brings the tube forward, while flexion of the neck brings its tip posteriorly.

Directional tubes, if used, allow the tube tip to be redirected

If the tube moves into the piriform recesses, lateral to the glottis, on advance (sometimes palpable in the neck), rotation of the tube can help to direct its tip medially, toward the laryngeal orifice.

Tube placement is confirmed in the usual fashion

Practicality: The technique is simple, portable, and easily affordable

BNTI may not be familiar, as it is not as popular as it once was, so it may require practice to understand how to direct head and neck position changes to facilitate intubation, as well as to learn to take cues from breath sounds

Indications: Anatomy that suggests difficult direct laryngoscopy

Need for intubation while preserving spontaneous ventilation

Inaccessibility of the oral cavity

Contraindications: Coagulopathy

Atresia of nares

Other causes of nasal cavity obstruction

Enlarged adenoids

Apneic patient (relative—procedure is less successful)

Upper airway trauma or obstruction

Facial or nasal trauma distorting nasal anatomy

Major head trauma

Suspected cervical spine injury

Complications: Turbinate injury or avulsion

Nasal hemorrhage (may be severe)

Gagging, choking, emesis

Aspiration of gastric contents

Misplaced ETT

Pharyngeal trauma

Laryngeal trauma

Placement of tube intracranially

REFERENCES:

1. Walls RM, Gurr DE, Kulkarni RG, et al. 6294 Emergency department intubations: second report of the ongoing National Emergency Airway Registry (NEAR) II study. *Ann Emerg Med* 2000;36:S51.

2. Dronen SC, Merigian DS, Hedges JR, et al. A comparison of blind nasotracheal and succinylcholine-assisted intubation in the poisoned patient. *Ann Emerg Med* 1987;16:650–652.

3. O'Connor RE, Megarget RE, Schnyder ME, et al. Paramedic success rates for blind nasotracheal intubation is improved with the use of an endotracheal tube with directional tip control. *Ann Emerg Med* 2000;36:328–332.

4. Steward DJ. *Manual of pediatric anesthesia*, 4th ed. New York: Churchill-Livingstone; 1995:88.

Blind Orotracheal Intubation

Concept: When tools for laryngoscopy are unavailable or unreliable, endotracheal tube (ETT) insertion may be facilitated by utilizing the fingers to guide the tube through the glottic opening (1,2), or by the use of a device designed to guide the tube through the oropharynx and into the glottis. Examples of the latter include the Williams airway intubator and the Berman intubating airway (3,4). In digital intubation, the index and long fingers of the nondominant hand are placed in the hypopharynx, feeling for the epiglottis anteriorly. They are then used to elevate and guide the tip of the styletted ETT just under the epiglottis, into the larynx. If reaching the epiglottis (at least) or glottis (optimally) is not possible due to short fingers or a deep larynx, the technique will be much less reliable, and essentially becomes a blind thrust towards the glottis. With the Williams or Berman guides, the device is inserted into the mouth of the anesthetized or unconscious patient, and the tube inserted blindly through it, to be guided towards the glottis.

Evidence: Little systematic testing of these techniques has been performed, nor are there useful comparative trials. Digital intubation is most likely to be utilized when highly unfavorable conditions for direct laryngoscopy exist, such as unavailability of a laryngoscope, copious amounts of blood or fluid in the airway, or the failure of all other techniques. It is more readily applicable in children than in adults, due to the short distance between the mouth and glottis. Case reports attest to its utility in difficult pediatric airway management (5,6). The Williams airway has been used to provide blind orotracheal intubation in the operating room in more than 300 cases, with a success rate of 80%(4).

a. Digital Intubation:

Preparation:

Same as for direct laryngoscopy (see Chapter 3)
Double gloving adds a measure of protection
Lubricate the stylet, place in ETT
Bend the ETT into a "field hockey stick" shape
The patient must be anesthetized and relaxed (to avoid trauma to the operator and to stimulate reflexes with coughing or emesis) or unconscious

Either sniffing position or neutral head position are acceptable
Pre-oxygenate, if time allows

Procedure (Figs. 16.1 to 16.4):

Stand beside the patient, facing the top of his/her head, with the nondominant hand closest to head
The index and long fingers of the nondominant hand are placed into the oropharynx
The epiglottis is palpated and lifted with the fingers
If epiglottis cannot be palpated, an assistant pulling on the tongue may elevate it to the point at which it can be palpated
The ETT is introduced, and guided between the two fingers
The dominant hand advances the tube along the groove between the index and long fingers, curving around the base of the tongue
While the index and long fingers guide the tube, it is advanced up under the epiglottis and into the glottis
The stylet is removed, ETT cuff inflated, and tube placement is confirmed
Alternatively, the index and long fingers of the nondominant hand can be inserted into the mouth with the curved, styletted tube held between them
As the fingers locate the glottis, the other (dominant) hand is used to advance the tube into the airway
The stylet is removed, ETT cuff inflated, and tube placement confirmed

b. Blind intubation through a Williams Airway intubator:

Preparation:

Same as for direct laryngoscopy (see Chapter 3)
Lubricate the ETT
Patient should be anesthetized or unconscious, pre-oxygenated, and in neutral position

Procedure (Figs. 16.5 to 16.7):

Williams airway intubator is inserted, its distal extent curving around the back of the tongue
Lubricated ETT is inserted through the intubator
Tube is gently advanced into the glottis

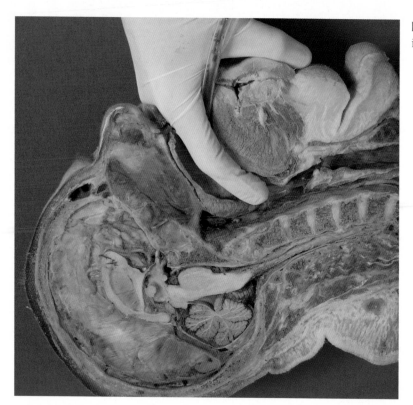

Figure 16.1 Digital intubation demonstrated in a cadaver specimen.

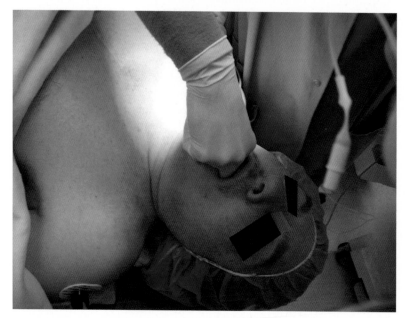

Figure 16.2 Fingers of nondominant hand, thrust behind tongue, lifting epiglottis.

Figure 16.3 ETT insertion, guided toward glottis by index and long fingers.

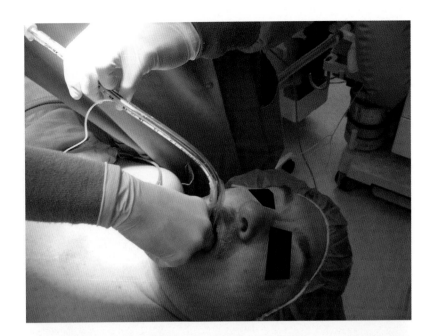

Figure 16.4 ETT advancing through glottis, guided by fingers.

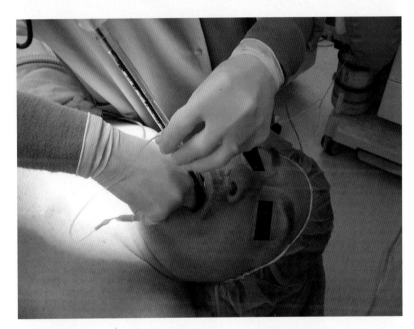

Figure 16.5 Berman and Williams airways, to facilitate blind orotracheal intubation.

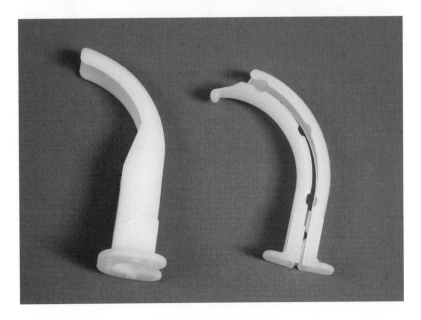

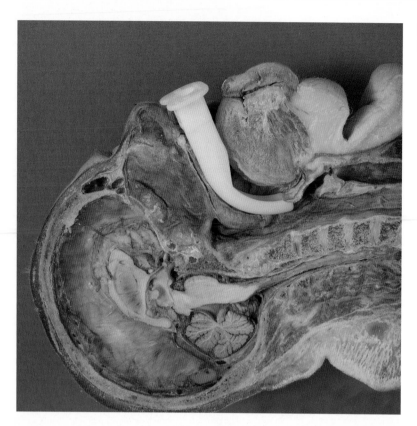

Figure 16.6 Placement of Williams airway in oropharynx in cadaver specimen.

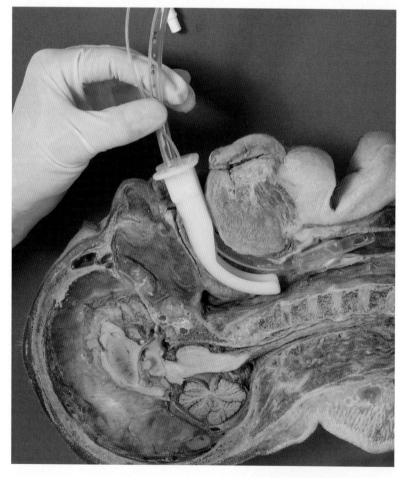

Figure 16.7 Advancing ETT through Williams airway blindly into glottis.

If resistance is met, the ETT is withdrawn and the airway intubator position modified, after which further attempts are conducted

Once placed, ETT cuff is inflated, and its position is confirmed in the usual fashion

Practicality: Simple, portable
Little or no cost
Unfamiliar to most—practice is desirable in patients or cadavers

Indications: Lack of laryngoscopy equipment
Failure of other techniques
Copious secretions or blood in airway
Patient in position that precludes direct laryngoscopy

Contraindications: Inability to palpate epiglottis (digital technique)
Inability to open the mouth
Infectious process or foreign body of airway
Disrupted larynx, or severe oropharyngeal trauma (unless no alternative means of managing the airway exists)

Conscious patient, or patient with intact airway reflexes

Complications: Misplacement of ETT
Trauma to pharynx or larynx from blind ETT insertion
Injury to hand of person intubating (digital technique)

REFERENCES:

1. Stewart RD. Tactile orotracheal intubation. *Ann Emerg Med* 1984;13:175—178.
2. Murphy MF, Hung OR. Blind digital intubation. In: Benumof JL, ed. *Airway management: principles and practice.* St. Louis: Mosby; 1996:277–281.
3. Berman RA. A method for blind oral intubation of the trachea or esophagus. *Anesth Analg* 1977;56:866–867.
4. Williams RT, Harrison RE. Prone tracheal intubation simplified using an airway intubator. *Can Anaesth Soc J* 1981;28: 288–289.
5. Hancock PJ, Peterson G. Finger intubation of the trachea in newborns. *Pediatrics* 1992;89:325–327.
6. Suetra PT, Gordon GJ. Digitally assisted tracheal intubation in a neonate with Pierre Robin syndrome. *Anesthesiology* 1993; 78:983–985.

Lightwands

Concept: The lightwand places a light source at the tip of the endotracheal tube (ETT). After the lightwand is threaded through the tube, the two are advanced blindly into the pharynx, aiming for the glottis. A "halo" of light visible over the front of the neck provides guidance for insertion of the tube and lightwand into the glottis, using gentle probing or rocking maneuvers. Transillumination of the larynx confirms that the tube is indeed being advanced into the airway.

In the late 1950s, Yamamura described transillumination for use in nasotracheal intubation (1). Use of the lighted stylet, or lightwand, has been well-described since then, as a blind technique in the setting of difficult laryngoscopy, as well as for routine airway management (2–4). Early commercial lightwands suffered from poor illumination and misdirection of the light, so that a darkened room was necessary to see the halo produced in the glottic area during insertion into the airway. The lamp switch was often placed in an awkward position. Further, an overly rigid stylet could cause retraction of the ETT out of the glottis when the lightwand was withdrawn (2). Newer models have improved upon the visibility of the light, as well as the ergonomics of the device (5). The Trachlight (Laerdal, Long Beach, CA), with its three-piece retractable wire lighted stylet, facilitates advancement of the lightwand-ETT and makes it unlikely that the ETT will be withdrawn from the trachea when the Trachlight device is pulled back. A locking device for the proximal portion of the ETT, and an adjustable length to accommodate different size tubes, also represent significant improvements of the Trachlite over earlier lighted stylets (5).

Evidence: In the operating room (OR), lighted stylet intubation has proven reliable and highly successful in both adults and children, in routine airway management and difficult airways (6). Ainsworth described intubation using the lighted stylet within 60 seconds in 200 patients under general anesthesia (4), whereas Weiss reported a series of 250 patients in whom he had 99% success in intubation utilizing this device (7). In 950 surgical patients, use of the Trachlite was compared to direct laryngoscopy for efficacy in tracheal intubation (5). Direct laryngoscopy was found to require more time, produce more complications, and result in a higher failure rate (3% vs.

1%). In 186 documented difficult airway patients, Hung utilized the Trachlight lighted stylet for intubation after induction of anesthesia with 99% success (8).

In the emergency department (ED), lighted stylets have also proven useful for airway management in facial trauma, and appear to facilitate intubation while preserving immobility of the cervical spine (9,10). In a series of 28 trauma patients with suspected cervical spine injury, the lightwand was employed for intubation with 100% success (11). The device has been adapted for nasotracheal intubation as well as orotracheal use (9). In prehospital care, Vollmer reported the use of the lighted stylet by emergency medicine residents in 24 patients with 88% success in less than 45 seconds (12).

The lightwand has been recommended for use in patients with known or potential cervical spine injury, as its use requires little or no motion of the cervical spine. Turkstra et al, evaluated cervical spine motion fluoroscopically in a crossover study of 36 healthy patients undergoing intubation with in-line immobilization (13). The authors compared the lighted stylet to intubation with the MacIntosh laryngoscope blade or use of a stylet during direct laryngoscopy, and found the least cervical spine motion occurred with the use of the lighted stylet for intubation. Inoue et al randomized 148 patients undergoing intubation during general anesthesia, with in-line immobilization of the cervical spine, to intubation with the lighted stylet or with the intubating laryngeal mask airway (LMA). The authors reported a 97% success with the Trachlight lightwand (Laerdal, Long Beach, CA), versus 73% for the intubating LMA, and concluded that the lightwand was more advantageous for orotracheal intubation in a population with known or potential cervical spine disorders (14).

The importance of the "bent length" (site of bending of the lighted stylet into a "hockey stick" shape) has recently been evaluated (15). Chen et al evaluated recommendations that the Trachlight device should optimally be bent 6.5 cm to 8.5 cm proximal to its distal tip (16). Based on clinical practice, the authors relate the optimal bent length to be the thyromental distance (TMD), that between the patient's thyroid cartilage prominence and the angle of the mandible. They report that for patients with TMD greater than 5.5 cm, the existing recommendations work well to optimize intubation success with the Trachlight device.

However, for smaller individuals, with TMD less than or equal to 5.5 cm, a bent length at the lower range of the recommendation (6.5 cm) should be utilized.

Preparation (Fig. 17.1):

Usual arrangements for orotracheal intubation (Chapter 3)

Lightwand prepared, lubricated, battery checked

Thread ETT over wand, until the distal tip with light bulb is at the end of the endtoracheal tube (but not protruding)

Ensure the proximal end of the ETT is held by the locking mechanism of the stylet, so that it does not slide up and down

Bend the lightwand-ETT into a "field hockey stick" configuration (90-degree to 120-degree bend proximal to cuff), 6.5 cm to 8.5 cm proximal to the tip of the lightwand

Anesthetized, pre-oxygenated patient, with airway reflexes controlled

Head in neutral position

Placing the illuminated stylet on the inside of the patient's cheek approximates the halo of light sought with laryngeal transillumination

Stand at the head of the patient

Procedure for Lightwand (Figs. 17.2 to 17.8):

Grasp/advance the mandible with nondominant hand

Insert lighted stylet (with light on) over back of tongue

Make attempts to advance into glottis, searching for opening by gently advancing the tube/stylet repeatedly towards the larynx in a "rocking" motion

If resistance is met, head extension, or jaw thrust may be helpful to facilitate glottic entry

Halo of light over larynx confirms glottic entry

Lack of halo, or halo in wrong site, provides cues to location of lightwand-ETT

When halo appears, advance the ETT, holding stylet in place

If transillumination cannot be visualized in larynx, consider reducing ambient light

Remove stylet, inflate ETT cuff, confirm ETT placement

Procedure for Trachlite Device (Figs. 17.9 and 17.10):

With Trachlite device, enter glottis in same fashion (using transillumination)

Retract wire stylet upon glottic entry

Advance tube and Trachlite further into glottis, until transillumination is noted in the lower neck, to level of sternal notch

Unlock the collar around the ETT adaptor

Advance the ETT off of the stylet

Grasp the ETT firmly

Remove the stylet, inflate ETT cuff, confirm tube placement

Practicality: Simple, portable

Trachlite is more complex; requires some practice and familiarity with its components

Affordable: the usual lightwand is $40 to $60, and the Trachlite is $300

Not a familiar technique; requires some training

Older models produce a poor halo and require a dark room

Very obese patients may render this technique ineffectual

Indications: Difficult laryngoscopy

Copious secretions or blood in airway

Routine intubation

Potential or known cervical spine injury in patient requiring airway management

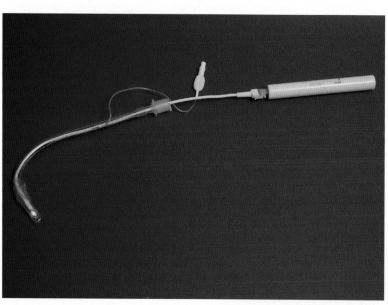

Figure 17.1 Lighted stylet with ETT.

Figure 17.2 Insertion of lightwand-ETT into oropharynx in cadaver specimen.

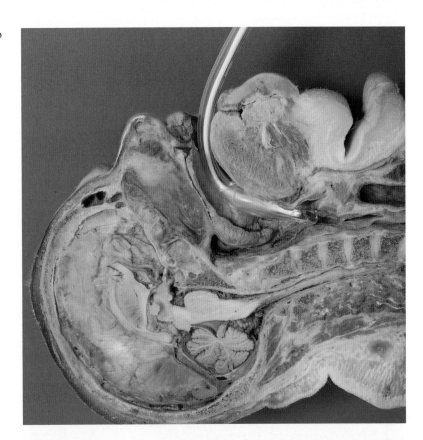

Figure 17.3 Lightwand-ETT approaching glottis.

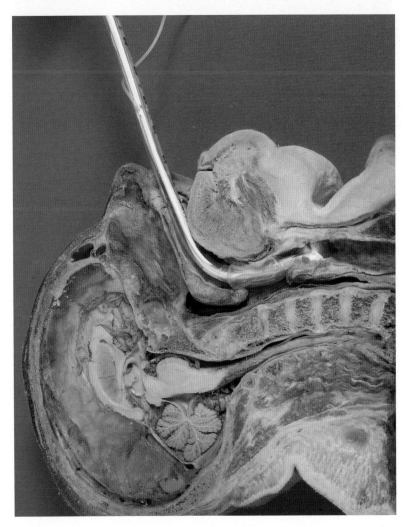

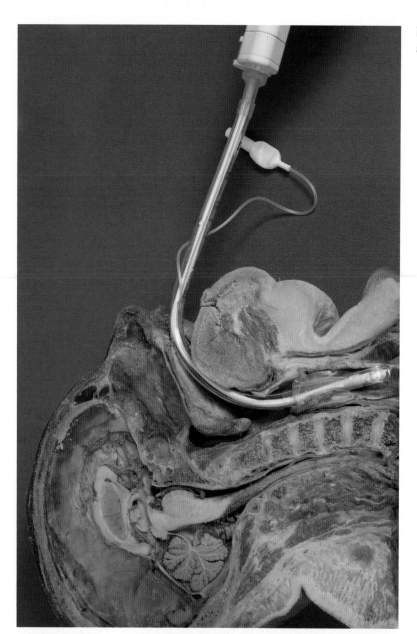

Figure 17.4 Lightwand-ETT advanced into airway.

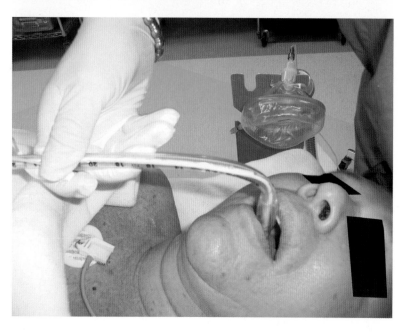

Figure 17.5 Insertion of lightwand-ETT.

Figure 17.6 The lightwand is advanced into the hypopharynx.

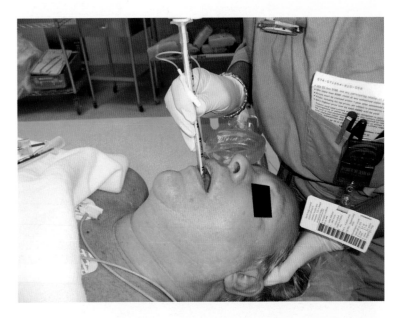

Figure 17.7 Halo of light produced by entry of lightwand-ETT into larynx.

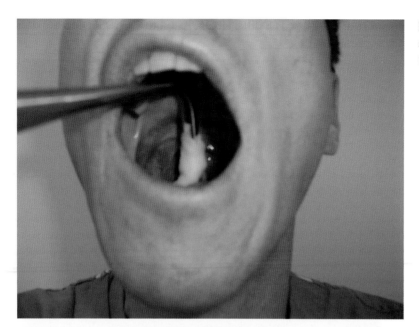

Figure 20.6 Krause forceps with a lidocaine-soaked pleget are placed in pyriform recess for superior laryngeal nerve block.

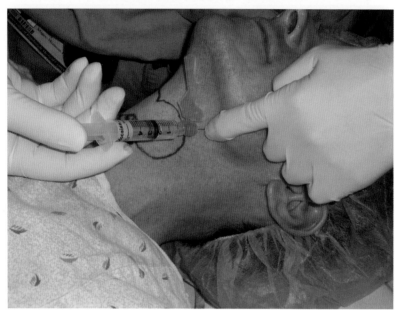

Figure 20.7 Superior laryngeal nerve block. Needle insertion occurs just medial and cephalad to the greater horn of the thyroid cartilage on each side.

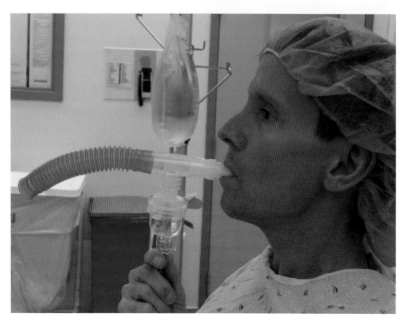

Figure 20.8 Lidocaine nebulization for laryngeal and tracheal anesthesia.

Figure 20.9 Transtracheal lidocaine injection conducted with a needle stick through the cricothyroid membrane. A catheter can also be placed for this purpose.

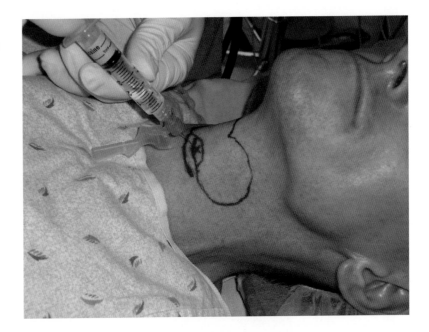

Procedure (for Orotracheal FOB Intubation)(Figs. 20.11 to 20.20):

Place oral Williams, Bermann, or Ovassapian airway, or have assistant use laryngoscope to elevate and compress tongue; a simple jaw thrust may also suffice

A mask with diaphragm, or anesthesia circuit with adaptor for FOB can be used with oral airway to maintain ventilation during FOB

Pass FOB through mask, bronchoscopy adaptor, or oral airway

Maintain scope tip in midline

Guide scope forward, curving the tip toward the glottis: upward and downward pressure with the thumb on the tip control lever curves the tip

Turn handle and scope tip as a unit; avoid twisting the insertion cord, which can break fibers

Visualize glottis through scope

Spray vocal cords with 1% lidocaine (2 mL) unless already topicalized with transtracheal injection or nebulization

Identify cords, advance scope between them

Advance scope tip until carina is in sight

Stabilize FOB, and advance ETT (or have assistant do this)

If resistance occurs, ETT bevel may be hung up on arytenoid cartilage or aryepiglottic fold: withdraw ETT slightly and turn 90 degrees counterclockwise, then attempt to advance gently

Figure 20.10 Williams airway inserted for FOB intubation in anesthetized patient.

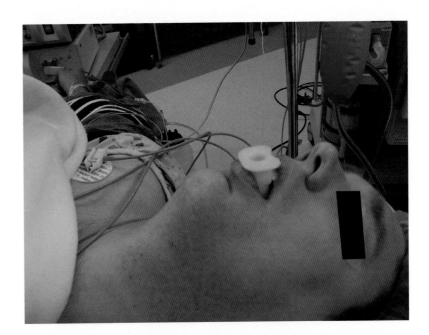

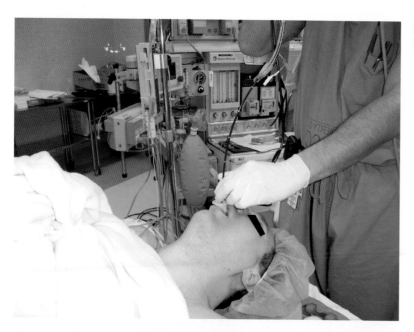

Figure 20.11 Insertion of FOB for oral intubation, from top of patient.

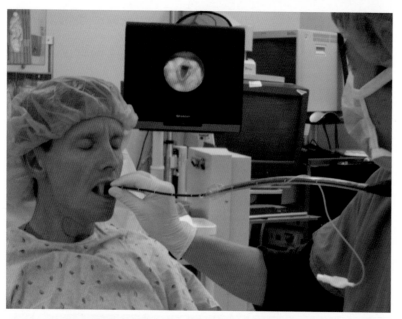

Figure 20.12 Insertion of FOB for oral intubation, from front of an awake, semi-recumbant patient.

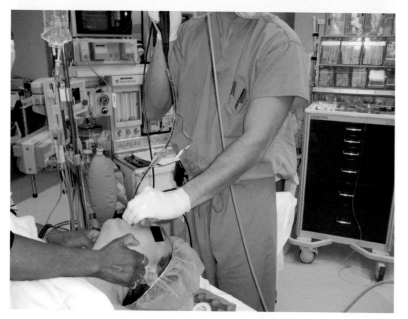

Figure 20.13 Jaw thrust during oral FOB insertion permits visualization of the glottis.

Figure 20.14 Oral ETT insertion over FOB.

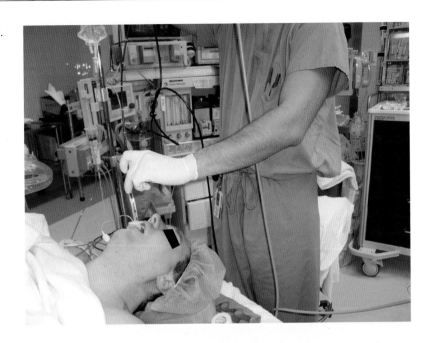

Figure 20.15 Oral FOB approach: insertion of ETT and FOB in cadaver specimen.

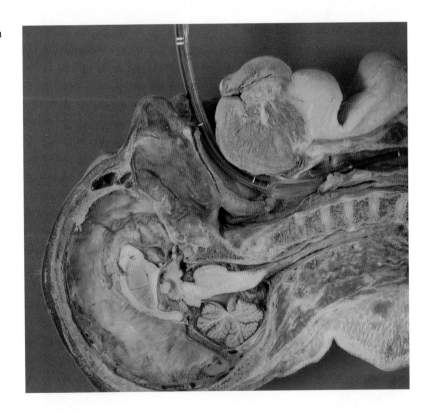

After tube passes into airway, remove FOB, visualize tracheal rings and ETT in airway on withdrawal

Confirm with detection of CO_2 and auscultation after scope is removed

Practicality: Unfamiliar and complex: requires considerable practice

Very expensive: scope, cart, and light source run more than $8,000

Awkward, multiple components, not easily portable

Battery-operated FOB reduces complexity and improves portability

Time-consuming: with patient preparation, awake FOB intubation may require more than 20 minutes

Requires logistic support for cleaning, maintenance

Indications: Predicted difficult intubation

Immobile cervical spine (halo, collar, in-line immobilization)

Difficult laryngoscopy, with preserved mask ventilation

Contraindications: Emergent intubation (due to time requirements)

Uncooperative patient (will not permit awake procedure)

Copious blood and secretions in airway

Inaccessibility of oral cavity

Procedure (for Nasal FOB Intubation) (Figs. 20.21 to 20.24):

Insert FOB into anesthetized, prepared nare

Advance along floor of nose

Visualize nasopharynx, curve tip of scope down toward glottis

Larynx should be in view

Advance tip of scope to glottis

Spray cords with 1% lidocaine 2 mL (unless already topicalized)

Advance tip of scope through glottic opening, confirm by noting tracheal rings

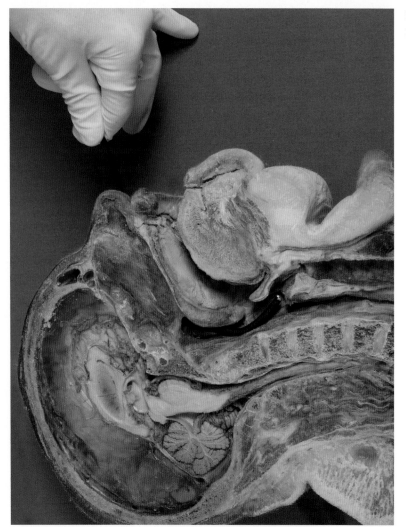

Figure 20.22 Insertion of FOB through nasal cavity in cadaver specimen.

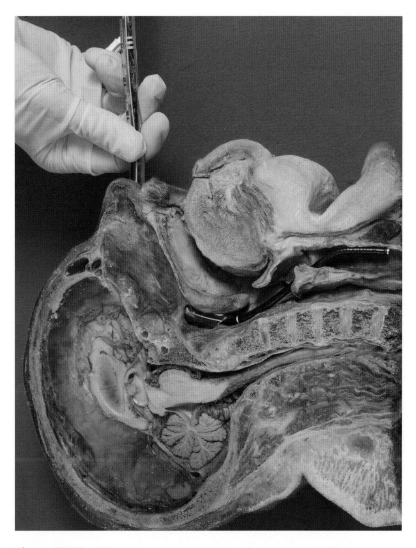

Figure 20.23 ETT advancement into nasopharynx over FOB.

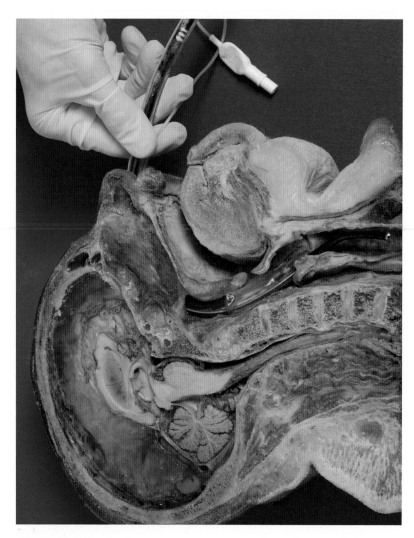

Figure 20.24 ETT placed over FOB into larynx.

Figure 20.25 Bevel of ETT "caught" on aryepiglottic fold during tube insertion, preventing intubation of trachea. Pulling the ETT back a few centimeters, rotating it 90 degrees counter-clockwise, and re-advancing usually solves this problem.

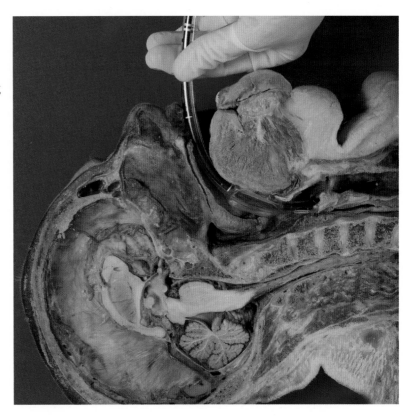

Continue to advance tip of scope until carina visualized

Stabilize scope and advance ETT over scope, into nose

Proceed with ETT insertion, through glottic opening

Alternatively, place ETT through nose to level of nasopharynx, then insert FOB, advancing into airway, followed by introduction of ETT

If ETT "hangs up" at larynx (Fig. 20.25), avoid force, and pull back ETT slightly, rotating it counter-clockwise 90 degrees, then re-advance gently

Confirm ETT is in airway as scope is withdrawn

Re-confirm ETT position with usual means

Indications: Inaccessibility of oral cavity
Cervical spine injury or immobility
Predicted difficult intubation

Contraindications: Emergent intubation (due to time required)
Coagulopathy or anticoagulation
Uncooperative patient
Copious blood or secretions in airway
Head or Facial Tumor

Complications of oral and nasal FOB intubation:
Inability to visualize airway (due to secretions, fogging, or tip of scope deviating laterally)

Misplacement of endotracheal tube

Trauma to larynx from insertion of ETT over the scope

Patient intolerance of awake procedure, usually due to insufficient topicalization of mucosa

Inability to pass ETT (occurs in up to 10% of cases), requiring smaller ETT to be used

Mainstem bronchus intubation

Patient hypoxia due to prolonged attempts, or failure to ventilate during attempts at intubation

Epistaxis (from nasal approach)

REFERENCES:

1. Ovassapian A, Wheeler M. Fiberoptic endoscopy-aided techniques. In: Benumof JL, ed. *Airway Management*. St. Louis: Mosby; 1996:282–319.
2. Ovassapian A, Doka JC, Romsa DE. Acromegaly. Use of a fiberoptic laryngoscope to avoid tracheostomy. *Anesthesiology* 1981;54:429–430.
3. Edens ET, Sia RL. Flexible fiberoptic endoscopy in difficult intubations. *Ann Otol Rhinol Laryngol* 1981;90:307–309.
4. Keenan MA, Stiles CM, Kaufman RL. Acquired laryngeal deviation associated with cervical spine disease in erosive, polyarticular arthritis. *Anesthesiology* 1983;58:441–449.
5. Ovassapian A, Yelian SJ, Dykes HM, et al. Fiberoptic nasotracheal intubation. *Anesth Analg* 1983;62:692–695.

6. Ovassapian A, Schreaker SC. Fiberoptic-aided bronchial intubation. *Semin Anesth* 1987;6:133–145.

7. Nakayama M, Kataoka N, Usui Y, et al. Techniques of nasotracheal intubation with the fiberoptic bronchoscope. *J Emerg Med* 1992;10:729–734.

8. Mulder Ds, Wallace DH, Woolhouse FM. The use of fiberoptic bronchoscope to facilitate endotracheal intubation following head and neck trauma. *J Trauma* 1975;15:638–640.

9. Benumof JL. Management of the difficult airway. *Anesthesiology* 1991;75:1087–1110.

10. Russell SH. Simultaneous use of two laryngoscopes. *Anaesth* 1993;48:918.

11. Ovassapian A. Fiberoptic airway endoscopy in critical care. In: Ovassapian A, ed. *Fiberoptic airway endoscopy in anesthesia and critical care.* New York: Raven Press; 1990:105–128.

12. Ovassapian A. Fiberoptic tracheal intubation with the esophageal-tracheal combitube in place. *Anesth Analg* 1993; 75:S385.

13. Finer NN, Muzyka D. Flexible endoscopic intubation of the neonate. *Pediatr Pulmonol* 1992;12:48–54.

14. Rucker RW, Lilva WJ, Worcester CC. Fiberoptic bronchoscopic nasotracheal intubation in children. *Chest* 1979;76: 56–62.

15. Baines DB, Goodrick MA, Beckenham EJ, et al. Fiberoptically guided endotracheal intubation in a child. *Anaesth Intens Care* 1989;17:354–355.

Rigid Fiberoptic Scopes

Concept: Rigid fiberoptic scopes permit indirect observation of the glottis, like their flexible counterparts. However, they are inserted into the hypopharynx to obtain a view of the glottis rather than into the airway. The endotracheal tube (ETT) is then inserted into the airway while visualizing its progress with the scope. Some types have a stylet onto which the ETT is loaded, others require freehand insertion. Several rigid fiberoptic scopes are available. The most familiar is the Bullard laryngoscope (ACMI; Southborough, MA) (Figs. 21.1 to 21.4). This device has a blade contour designed to match the anatomy of the upper airway, which mounts on a standard laryngoscope handle. It features a fiberoptic bundle which lies on the posterior aspect of the blade and ends quite close to the end of the blade. It also possesses a working channel for introduction of local anesthetics, suction, or oxygen insufflation. To intubate with the Bullard, the operator inserts the scope into the hypopharynx in an anesthetized patient, and advances the blade into position cephalad to the glottis. This affords an excellent view of the larynx. The ETT can then be pushed forward off the stylet (or placed freehand), into the glottis, while observing it through the instrument. Other available rigid scopes include the Upsherscope (Mercury Medical, Clearwater, FL) (Fig. 21.5) and the WuScope (Achi Corporation, San Jose, CA) (Fig. 21.6).

Evidence: Of the available rigid fiberoptic scopes, the Bullard has been the most extensively evaluated. This device appears to be safe and effective for airway management in the patient with a potential cervical spine injury (1). Watts compared the time required for intubation and the degree of cervical extension utilizing the Bullard scope versus that for direct laryngscopy, both with and without in-line cervical immobilization, in patients under general anesthesia (2). The degree of spine extension and the time to intubate were similar, except when cervical immobilization was imposed, at which time the average duration required for intubation with the Bullard scope was significantly prolonged, ranging from 25 seconds to 40 seconds. However, Schulman reported in a randomized trial in 50 patients under anesthesia that, in comparing the Bullard scope to a flexible fiberscope during in-line cervical immobilization, intubation was significantly easier to accomplish and required less time with the rigid apparatus (3). The

Bullard scope has proven useful for management of normal and difficult pediatric airways (4).

The Upsherscope, a relatively new rigid scope incorporating a C-shaped steel blade with the enclosed fiberoptic bundles and an intubation channel, proved to have no advantage over direct laryngoscopy in enabling intubation in a group of 300 patients randomly assigned to airway management in the operating room (OR) by either technique (5). In fact, the authors reported a 15% failure rate with the Upsherscope, compared to 3% with direct laryngoscopy. Yet another rigid scope, the WuScope, was compared to direct laryngoscopy in 87 patients randomized to either form of airway management during in-line cervical immobilization to simulate potential cervical injury during anesthesia for elective surgery (6). The authors found similar rates of intubation success, but longer intubation times and lower glottic visualization scores using the WuScope.

Preparation for Bullard Laryngoscope Intubation:

Typical preparation for direct laryngoscopy (see Chapter 3)
Administer an antisialagogue 15 minutes to 20 minutes before procedure
Assemble laryngoscope to fiberoptic light source handle, and attach nonmalleable wire stylet (if stylet is to be used)
For adults over 6 feet tall, a plastic blade extender should be used (this snaps onto the Bullard laryngoscope blade, lengthening it)
Check scope light intensity, optics, view
Use anti-fog solution on lens
Pre-oxygenate and anesthetize patient in neutral position (or, with proper airway anesthesia and sedation, the patient can undergo awake intubation)
Lubricate ETT and load on the Bullard's stylet (distal end of stylet should project through the Murphy eye of tube)
Attach oxygen tubing to Luer-lock fitting on proximal end of scope to insufflate oxygen during intubation attempts, if desired

Procedure (Figs. 21.2 to 21.4):

Stand at head of bed, open mouth with right hand
Insert Bullard scope with left hand, guide the blade

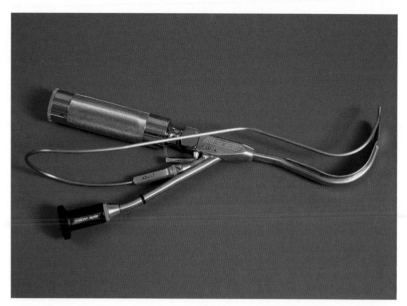

Figure 21.1 The Bullard laryngoscope.

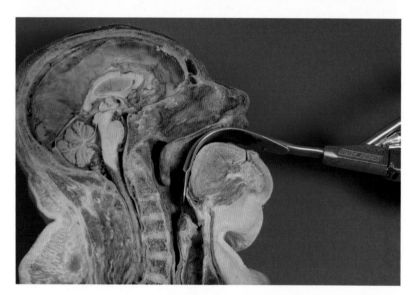

Figure 21.2 Bullard scope positioned in hypopharynx in cadaver specimen (stylet removed for clarity).

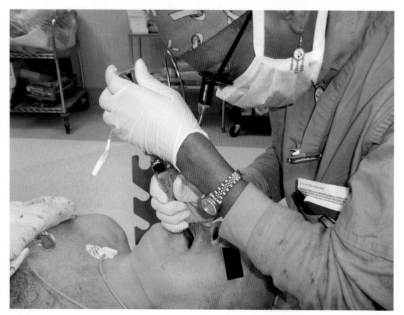

Figure 21.3 Optimizing the view of the glottis with the Bullard scope requires lifting the epiglottis with the blade.

Figure 21.4 View through the Bullard scope, with tip of ETT seen on right of image, poised to enter the glottis as it is advanced off of the attached stylet.

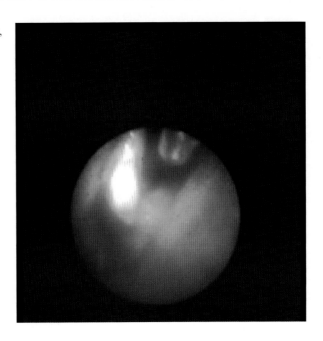

Figure 21.5 The Upsherscope. (Courtesy of Mercury Medical, Clearwater, FL.)

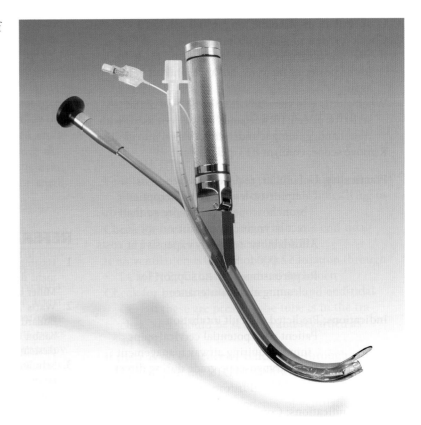

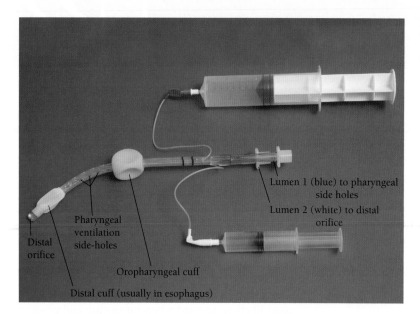

Pharyngeal
ventilation
side-holes

Distal
orifice

Oropharyngeal cuff

Distal cuff (usually in esophagus)

Lumen 1 (blue) to pharyngeal
side holes

Lumen 2 (white) to distal
orifice

Figure 22.1 The esophageal tracheal combitube (ETC). Note two tubes with two cuffs, two pilot balloons and two lumens.

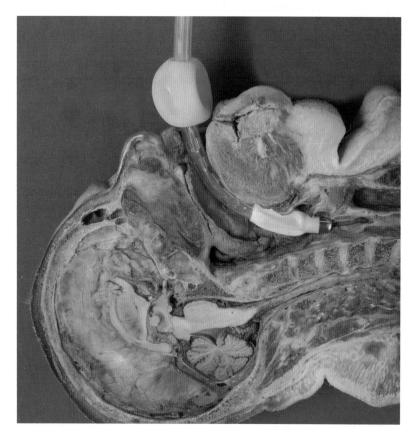

Figure 22.2 ETC inserted into pharynx in cadaver specimen.

Figure 22.3 ETC advanced into esophagus.

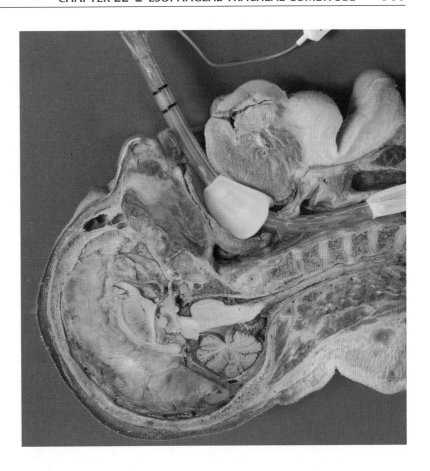

Figure 22.4 Cuffs of ETC inflated. Note proximity of pharyngeal side holes to glottic opening, and seal provided by distal and proximal balloons.

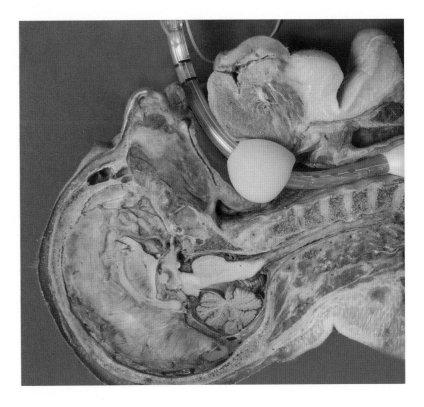

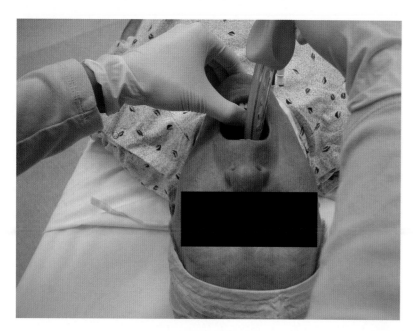

Figure 22.5 To insert the ETC, the head is placed in neutral position and the mandible pulled forward by grasping the lower teeth and chin while opening the mouth simultaneously. The ETC is then inserted through the pharynx into the esophagus (rarely, the trachea) blindly, until the black bands visible on the external surface of the device are aligned on either side of the incisors.

Indications: Inability to intubate or ventilate
May be used in lieu of laryngoscopic intubation by prehospital providers who are not skilled or trained in endotracheal intubation
Lack of a laryngoscope, when airway control is necessary

Contraindications: Alert or responsive patient
Supraglottic obstruction (tumor, foreign body)
Esophageal injury or disease
Inaccessibility of oral cavity
Laryngeal or pharyngeal trauma

Complications: Esophageal and pharyngeal trauma, including significant lacerations, has been described (7,8)
Failure to ventilate due to malposition

REFERENCES:

1. Frass M, Johnson JC, Atheton GL, et al. Esophageal tracheal combitube for emergency intubation. *Resuscitation* 1989;18: 95–102.
2. Rumball CJ, MacDonald D. The PTL, combitube, laryngeal mask and oral airway. *Prehosp Emerg Care* 1997;1:1–10.
3. Wissler RN. Esophageal tracheal combitube. *Anesth Rev* 1993; 20:147–152.
4. Staudinger MD, Brugger S, Watschinger B. Emergency intubation with the combitube. *Ann Emerg Med* 1993;22:1573–1575.
5. Frass M. Mechanical ventilation with the esophageal tracheal combitube in the intensive care unit. *Arch Emerg Med* 1987;4: 219–223.
6. Frass M. Ventilation with the esophageal tracheal combitube in cardiopulmonary resuscitation. *Chest* 1988;93:781–786.
7. Vezina D, Lessard MR, Bussieres J, et al. Complications associated with the use of the esophageal-tracheal combitube. *Can J Anaesth* 1998;45:76–80.
8. Richards CF. Piriform sinus perforation during esophageal-tracheal combitube placement. *J Emerg Med* 1999;17:37–39.

23

Laryngeal Mask Airway

Concept: The laryngeal mask airway (LMA) (Laryngeal Mask of North America, San Diego, CA) has been in widespread use by anesthesiologists in Europe since the 1980s, when it was developed by Dr. AIJ Brain (1). It is utilized worldwide in the operating room (OR) to ensure airway patency during general anesthesia. The device is available in both reusable and disposable forms (Figs. 23.1 and 23.2), and is comprised of a tube attached to an ovoid mask that is placed in the hypopharynx, and advanced to cover the glottic opening. When inflated, the cuff of this mask provides a seal around the glottic aperture (2). However, this seal is inadequate at high peak inspiratory pressures, and leakage of inspiratory gases is manifest, especially when pressures begin to exceed 30 cm H_2O. In elective settings, spontaneous breathing (as opposed to positive pressure ventilation) is preferred with the use of this device, but it can be used safely and effectively for positive pressure ventilation if tidal volumes and peak inspiratory pressures are kept low (tidal volume should not exceed 8 mL/kg and peak inspiratory pressures should be limited to 20 cm H_2O). The LMA is manufactured in many sizes, ranging from those for neonates to those for large adults. In adults, the usual range of sizes is 3, 4, and 5. Multiple manufacturers have now begun to offer similar devices.

Because the LMA does not provide an intra-tracheal seal, regurgitation and aspiration are potential risks of its use. This prompted the development of a version of the device that incorporates a gastric port to allow decompression of the stomach after insertion. The Proseal LMA (LMA of North America, San Diego, CA) (Fig. 23.3) was designed to separate the respiratory and gastrointestinal tracts, and provide higher airway sealing pressures, thus allowing dependable positive pressure ventilation. The Proseal LMA can be somewhat more challenging to insert than the standard LMA device, due to its larger size and different conformation. This device can be placed freehand, or with an introducer device. Both the standard LMA and the Proseal LMA devices can be over-inflated, with resultant mucosal injury (5). Ideally, a manometer should be used to gauge the correct pressure of inflation.

Evidence: The LMA is effective for ventilation in the operating room during many types of elective surgical cases (1,2). The LMA has also been utilized as an emergency ventilation adjunct in a variety of circumstances (2–4). It can be used effectively as a "bridge" to fiberoptic intubation, because a size 6.0 endotracheal tube (ETT) (or 7.0 in the size 5 LMA) may be passed through the LMA and into the glottis, while the lumen of the device effectively guides the fiberscope to the laryngeal opening (4,6). The LMA has proven useful as a both an alternative to bag-valve-mask (BVM) ventilation in cardiopulmonary arrest and as a rescue device in difficult airway management. Among intensive care nurses, Martin found that the LMA proved easier to use, and provided superior tidal volumes with less likelihood of airway obstruction, than BVM ventilation with or without an oral airway (7). When untrained volunteers were assessed for the ability to ventilate patients under general anesthesia, Alexander described marked improvement in success of ventilation and oxygenation when the LMA was used, compared with BVM ventilation (8). He reported a 43% rate of failure to ventilate effectively with the latter device, whereas the LMA was successful in all but 13% of cases. Likewise, Smith found that anesthetists were better able to maintain oxygen saturation and a patent airway in 64 patients under general anesthesia randomly assigned to ventilation using the LMA as opposed to a face mask (9).

In an evaluation of the utility of LMA for prehospital care, Pennant described placement of LMA by paramedics in 100% of cases in less than 40 seconds, whereas ETT placement required more than twice that long and resulted in 31% misplacement (10). Davies described placement of an ETT or LMA in a mannequin model by paramedics with little training: 94% of LMA insertions were successful, compared with only 51% of ETT insertions (11).

The LMA has been well established for effectiveness during difficult airway management in the OR (3,4,6). Experienced practitioners can usually insert the LMA within 20 seconds, with a success rate of 98% (12). Parnet described the use of LMA as the adjunct of first choice by academic anesthesiologists facing difficult intubation or difficult ventilation situations in 17 cases over 2 years, with a 94% success rate, whereas other modalities were significantly less successful (13). Very few reports exist describing failure of an LMA in a cannot-intubate, cannot-ventilate (failed airway) situation (14). Thus the considerable experience with the LMA in unexpectedly difficult airway management in the OR substantiates its use when emergent

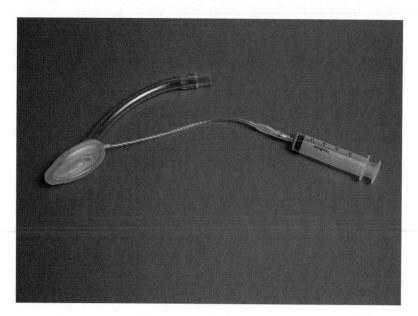

Figure 23.1 LMA Unique (disposable).

ventilation is required in other settings, such as the emergency department (ED) or intensive care unit (ICU), because it can be inserted so quickly and with a high expectation of success (15). Its use may allow progression to a more definitive airway, whether translaryngeal or surgical, in a controlled and orderly manner, as opposed to a frenetic procedure in a severely hypoxemic patient. Given its utility in emergency circumstances, the LMA has become the intervention of choice for the cannot-intubate, cannot-ventilate situation in the operating room, as directed by the 2003 difficult airway management guidelines of the American Society of Anesthesiology (16).

A variety of case reports of gastric aspiration related to LMA use have been published (17). A number of these patients had predispositions to regurgitation due to obesity,

surgical position, or emergency procedures. In a large meta-analysis of the literature, Brimacombe concluded that the incidence of reported aspiration of gastric contents with the use of the LMA device was no higher than that reported with the use of the endotracheal tube, in the elective surgical patient (18).

The Proseal LMA provides a higher sealing pressure than the standard LMA, facilitating mechanical ventilation, and allows passage of a gastric tube to decompress the stomach, offering a measure of protection against aspiration (19). Like the LMA, it has proven effective in management of the difficult airway and for rescue in cannot-intubate, cannot-ventilate situations (20). Failure of placement with the device may be as high as 4% (21). Proseal LMA is offered in two pediatric sizes (2 and 3), and

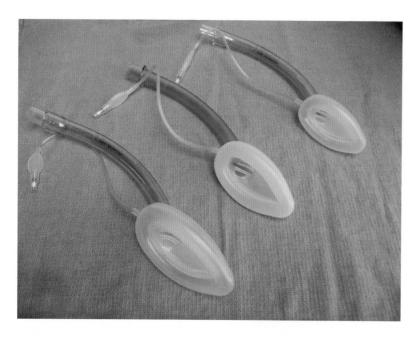

Figure 23.2 LMA Unique in sizes 3, 4, 5 (for patients less than 50 kg, 50 kg to 70 kg, and greater than 70 kg, respectively). Note the aperture bars at the distal end of the airway tube, to prevent tube occlusion by the epiglottis.

Figure 23.3 Proseal LMA (note gastric port). (Courtesy of LMA of North America, San Diego, CA.)

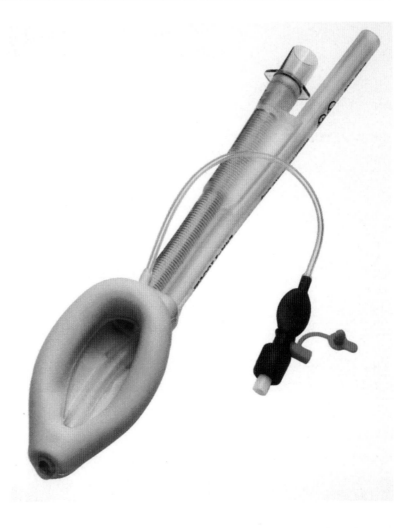

has been demonstrated to provide a more effective seal with less gastric insufflation than the standard LMA in a population of thirty children (10 kg to 21 kg) (22).

Preparation:

Preparation for direct laryngscopy (see Chapter 3)
Estimate size of LMA necessary, based on patient size, weight (see Table 23.1)
Lubricate dorsal (top) surface of LMA
Check integrity of cuff, and deflate completely
Anesthetized, or unconscious patient in neutral position
Pre-oxygenation is optimal (but in cannot-intubate, cannot-ventilate scenarios will be impossible)

Procedure for insertion of laryngeal mask airway (Figs. 23.4 to 23.12):

Open mouth, extend head with nondominant hand
Slide the dorsal surface of the LMA along hard palate of the patient
Hold the device like a pencil in the right hand, with index finger between the tube and mask at its base
Use index finger to guide LMA into pharynx, initially exerting force cephalad, against the hard palate

Table 23.1

LMA Sizes and Inflation Volumes

Size of LMA Device	Weight of Patient	Maximum Inflation Volume (mL)*
1	Infants to 5 kg	4
1.5	5–10 kg	7
2	10–20 kg	10
2.5	20–30 kg	14
3	30–50 kg	20
4	50–70 kg	30
5	70–100 kg	40
6 (LMA classic only)	>100 kg	50

* The manufacturer recommends that cuff pressures not exceed 60 cm H_2O. In sizing, the largest size that fits readily into the patient's pharynx should be chosen, and inflated until there is no leak at 20 cm H_2O inspiratory pressure.

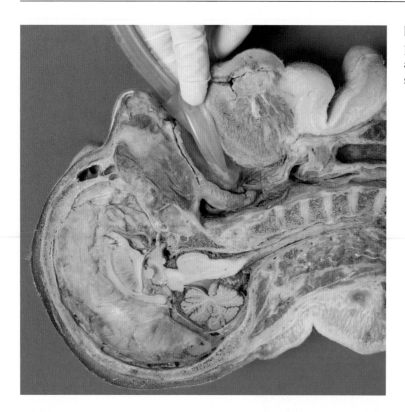

Figure 23.4 LMA insertion: dorsal surface pressed against the hard palate, as LMA is advanced toward pharynx, in cadaver specimen.

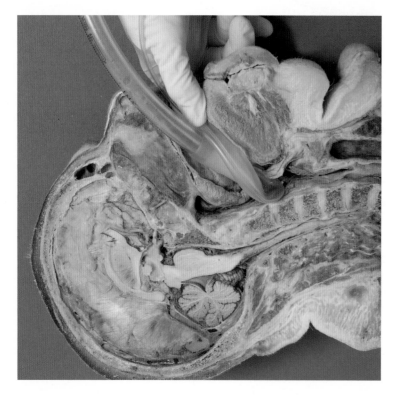

Figure 23.5 LMA is advanced into the pharynx.

Figure 23.6 LMA in place over larynx.

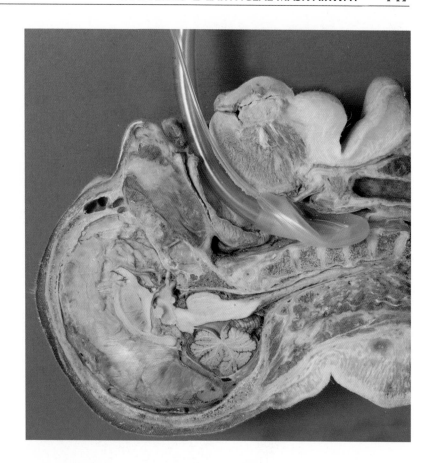

Figure 23.7 The cuff is now inflated to create a seal around the larynx.

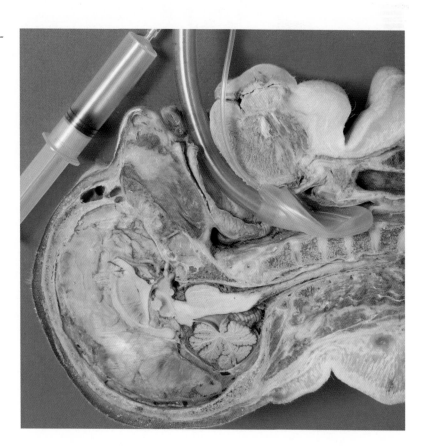

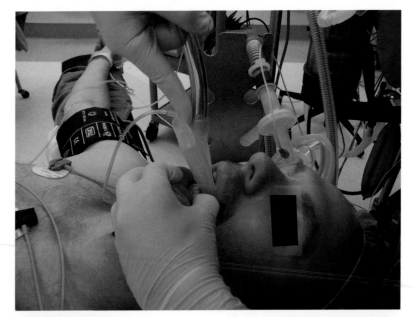

Figure 23.8 Preparing to insert the LMA.

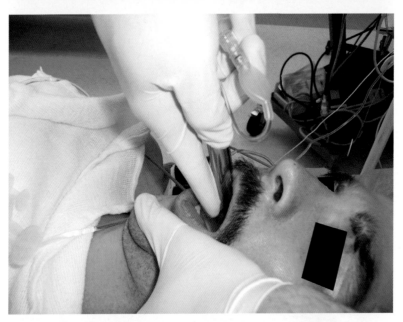

Figure 23.9 Insertion of LMA in elective situation in OR. Note position of index finger to guide the device along the hard palate and into the hypopharynx.

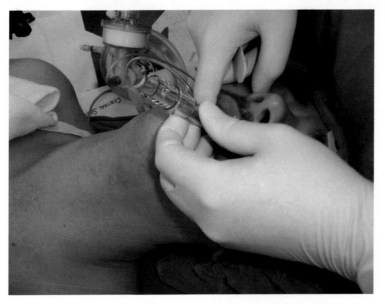

Figure 23.10 Continue insertion until resistance is met as LMA seats in hypopharynx.

Figure 23.11 LMA sliding along hard palate as it is introduced toward the pharynx.

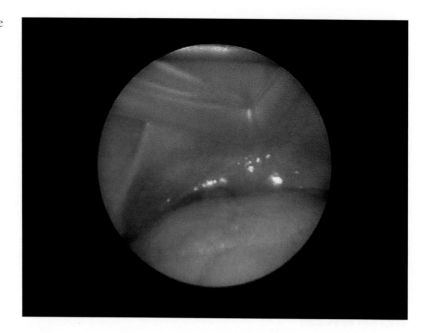

The index finger continues to exert force, assisting in the acute bend that the mask and tube must negotiate to seat in the hypopharynx
Advance LMA into hypopharynx until resistance is felt
Inflate the cuff (volume of air depends on the LMA size)
Confirm chest rise, breath sounds, end-tidal carbon dioxide ($ETCO_2$)
Secure the device

Practicality: Inexpensive
Portable and simple
Relatively unfamiliar for those not using it routinely; requires use and practice for facility

Indications: Routine airway in OR
Difficult laryngoscopy
Difficult ventilation
First choice in OR for cannot-intubate, cannot-ventilate scenario
Planned bridge to fiberscopic intubation

Contraindications: Severe upper airway obstruction
Inaccessibility of oral cavity
Full stomach, or potential for gastric regurgitation (this applies to elective use of the device)
Planned positive pressure ventilation, if peak airway pressures are likely to exceed 20 cm H_2O

Figure 23.12 Bronchoscopic view inside lumen of LMA showing epiglottis just beyond grill at the end of LMA lumen (epiglottis not folded down).

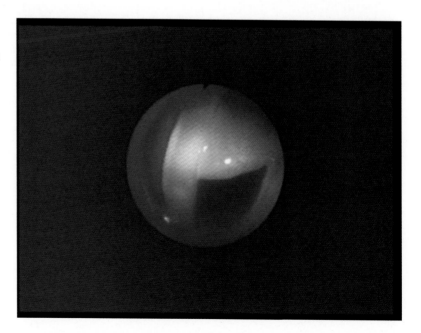

Complications: Regurgitation/aspiration of gastric contents

Failure to seal over the glottis, with inadequate ventilation

Gas leak at high peak inspiratory pressures (about 30% of tidal volume is lost at inspiratory pressures greater than 30 cm H_2O)

May stimulate swallowing, cough, or hiccups when inserted

Laryngospasm

Pharyngeal trauma during blind insertion

Nerve injury due to compression (CN IX, X, XII)

Overinflation of cuff with pharyngeal mucosal injury

REFERENCES:

1. Brain AIJ. The laryngeal mask airway. *Br J Anaesth* 1983;55: 801–804.

2. Pennant JH. Laryngeal mask airway. *Anesthesiology* 1993;79: 144–163.

3. Benumof JL. Use of the laryngeal mask airway to facilitate fiberoptic bronchoscopic intubation. *Anesth Analg* 1992;74: 313–315.

4. Benumof JL. Laryngeal mask airway and the ASA difficult airway algorithm. *Anesthesiology* 1996;84:686–699.

5. Keller C, Brimacombe J. Mucosal pressure and oropharyngeal leak pressure with the ProSeal versus laryngeal mask airway in anesthetized, paralyzed patients. *Br J Anaesth* 2000; 85:262–266.

6. Heath ML, Allagain J. Intubation through the laryngeal mask. *Anesthesiology* 1991;46:545–548.

7. Martin PD, Cyna AM, Hunter WAH, et al. Training nursing staff in airway management for resuscitation. *Anesthesiology* 1993;48:33–37.

8. Alexander R, Hodgson P, Lomax D, et al. A comparison of the laryngeal mask airway and Guedel airway, bag and face-mask for manual ventilation following formal training. *Anesthesiology* 1993;48:231–234.

9. Smith I, White PF. Use of the laryngeal mask airway as an alternative to a face mask in outpatient arthroscopy. *Anesthesiology* 1992;47:850–855.

10. Pennant JH, Walker MB. Comparison of the endotracheal tube and laryngeal mask in airway management by para-medical personnel. *Anesth Analg* 1992;74:531–534.

11. Davies PRF, Tighe SQM, Greenslade GL, et al. Laryngeal mask airway and endotracheal tube insertion by unskilled personnel. *Lancet* 1990;336:977–979.

12. Brimacombe JR, Berry A. Mallampati class and laryngeal mask airway insertion. *Anaesth* 1993;48:347–351.

13. Parnet JL, Colonna-Romano P, Horrow JC, et al. The laryngeal mask airway reliably provides rescue ventilation in cases of unanticipated difficult tracheal intubation along with difficult mask ventilation. *Anesth Analg* 1998;87: 661–665.

14. Patel SK, Whitten CW, Ivy R, et al. Failure of the laryngeal mask airway: an undiagnosed laryngeal carcinoma. *Anesth Analg* 1998;86:438–439.

15. Pollock CV Jr. The laryngeal mask airway: a comprehensive review for the emergency physician. *J Emerg Med* 2001;20: 53–56.

16. Caplan RA, Benumof JL, Berry FA, et al. Practice guidelines for management of the difficult airway: an updated report by the ASA task force on management of the difficult airway. *Anesthesiology* 2003;98:1269–1277.

17. Keller C, Brimacombe J, Bittersohl J, et al. Aspiration and the laryngeal mask airway: three cases and a review of the literature. *Br J Anaesth* 2004;93:579–582.

18. Brimacombe JR, Berry A. The incidence of aspiration associated with the laryngeal mask airway: a meta-analysis of published literature. *J Clin Anesth* 1995;7:297–303.

19. Brimacombe J, Keller C. The Proseal laryngeal mask airway. *Anesth Clin NA* 2002;20:871–891.

20. Cook TM, Silsby J, Simpson TP. Airway rescue in acute upper airway obstruction using a Proseal laryngeal mask airway and an Airtree catheter: A review of the Proseal laryngeal mask airway in management of the difficult airway. *Anesthesia* 2005;60:1129–1136.

21. Gaitini LA, Vaida SJ, Somri M. A randomized controlled trial comparing the Proseal Laryngeal Mask Airway with the Laryngeal Tube Suction in mechanically ventilated patients. *Anesthesiology* 2004;101:316–320.

22. Goldmann K, Jakob C. Size 2 Proseal laryngeal mask airway: a randomized, crossover investigation with the standard laryngeal mask airway in pediatric patients. *Br J Anaesth* 2005; 94:385–389.

24

Intubating Laryngeal Mask Airway

Concept: The intubating LMA (ILMA) (Fastrach, LMA of North America, San Diego, CA) is a derivation of the LMA that facilitates blind endotracheal intubation. The device has several features that distinguish it from the standard laryngeal mask device. The intubating laryngeal mask consists of a soft mask that fits over the larynx, attached to a rigid stainless steel tube. Attached to the tube is a handle to facilitate insertion, and the lumen has a larger internal diameter than the standard adult LMA. This tube admits a flexible, reinforced endotracheal tube (ETT) specifically manufactured for this laryngeal mask. The device comes in three sizes for adults (3, 4, and 5), all of which can admit a range of ETT sizes, up to size 8.0. Other manufacturers have begun to offer similar devices, such as the Intubating Laryngeal Airway (ILA)(Mercury Medical, Clearwater, FL). The ILA also provides ready intubation through the device, but does not have the steel barrel or handle.

A new version of the ILMA features a view screen that is attached to the laryngeal mask after it is inserted and ventilation is established (C-trach, LMA of North America, San Diego, CA). This device provides both a light source and imaging capability, so that blindly advancing the ETT is no longer necessary. Instead, the provider can observe the approach of the ETT towards, and into, the airway.

Evidence: The ILMA device has proven useful for managing the difficult airway in a variety of settings. The enormous popularity of the LMA in Europe and other areas around the world has led to ready acceptance of the ILMA. In Australia, Agro described its use in 110 patients slated for general anesthesia, with 95% success (1). However, the authors encountered resistance to ETT insertion, which required some form of adjustment, in 60% of patients. The average time required for the authors to intubate patients was 79 seconds. In a multicenter study from the UK, Baskett assessed the efficacy of the ILMA in intubation of 500 patients undergoing general anesthesia, with 95% success in ventilation through the mask portion of the device (2). The authors had 80% intubation success on the first attempt, with 4% of patients requiring three attempts, and an overall failure rate of 4%. Brain used the ILMA in 150 patients undergoing general anesthesia, with

successful ventilation of all patients (3). In half of patients, resistance to ETT insertion through the device occurred, requiring one of several described "adjusting maneuvers" before intubation was accomplished. The study included 13 patients with potential or known difficult airway anatomy, all of whom were intubated successfully. A slate of four different adjusting maneuvers was presented, based upon the level at which resistance to the ETT is encountered (3).

In 38 patients with known difficult airway anatomy (based on patient history or physical exam), Joo assessed the utility of the ILMA compared with awake intubation with the fiberoptic bronchoscope (FOB) (4). All awake FOB attempts were successful, but only half of patients could be intubated blindly with the ILMA. The other half required use of a bronchoscope, and 10% required involvement of a second operator to place the ETT. In another evaluation of this device in patients with known or suspected difficult airways, Ferson et al evaluated the utility of the ILMA in 257 patients: 78% after induction of anesthesia, and 20% awake, with topical anesthesia (in 2% of cases, patients were unconscious and no anesthetic was provided)(5). The authors were able to ventilate these patients successfully in 100% of cases, and ETT insertion was accomplished blindly in 96.5% of the 200 in whom it was attempted (the remainder were intubated with FOB, utilizing the ILMA as an introducer device), 75% on the first attempt.

In a study of the efficacy of the ILMA in obese patients, Combes et al found that the device required less adjusting maneuvers and fewer attempts at blind placement than in lean subjects, with similar overall intubation success rates (96% versus 94%, respectively) (6). Among anesthetized patients placed in in-line cervical immobilization to simulate suspected cervical spine trauma, Komatsu et al found that the ILMA was simpler and quicker to insert than another supraglottic ventilation device, the laryngeal tube, and allowed ventilation with larger tidal volumes (7). Case series suggest that this device can be used safely in the patient with cervical spine injuries or disorder (8,9).

Less data exist related to use of the ILMA in emergency intubation, outside the operating room (OR). Asai, simulating trauma resuscitation with manual in-line

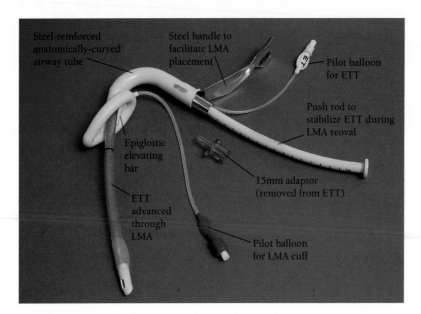

Figure 24.1 The intubating LMA, and its push rod and dedicated ETT.

immobilization of the cervical spine in anesthetized patients, evaluated the ILMA for intubation in 40 patients (10). The ILMA was used in conjunction with FOB to ensure correct placement, and this tandem was compared to direct laryngoscopy with use of a bougie. The authors reported 85% success of intubation with the ILMA under these circumstances, but less than half of the patients in the laryngoscopy-bougie group were successfully intubated with these conditions. Rosenblatt reported three cases of successful intubation with the ILMA in patients in whom direct laryngoscopy had failed in the emergency department (ED) (11). The authors commented of the ILMA that "proficiency in its use requires practice under controlled conditions," and suggested that "the emergency physician seek out elective practice" before it is used for airway management under emergent circumstances.

Preparation (Figs. 24.1 and 24.2):

Preparation for direct laryngoscopy (see Chapter 3)
Estimate size of ILMA necessary for patient, based on size and weight
Lubricate both ILMA (dorsal cuff) and the reinforced ETT
Check cuff of both ILMA and ETT
Place ETT through LMA to ensure smooth function and lubrication
Anesthetized, pre-oxygenated patient, in neutral or sniffing position

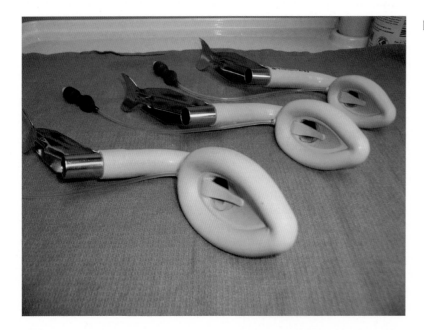

Figure 24.2 ILMA in three sizes for adults.

Procedure (Figs. 24.3 to 24.19):

Open mouth, place the ILMA into the pharynx, utilizing the handle to rotate the mask into the hypopharynx, until resistance is felt

Inflate ILMA cuff, confirm optimal ventilation

Stabilize ILMA, and insert ETT (without 15 mm connector) through it with longitudinal black stripe facing cephalad

When black band on ETT (15 cm) reaches the proximal lumen of LMA device, the tip of the ETT is at the epiglottic elevating bar (distal end of LMA lumen)

Advance ETT, lifting gently on the handle of the ILMA device

If resistance is encountered, note depth, and utilize adjusting maneuvers as necessary (see Table 24.1)

When ETT advances smoothly with no resistance, inflate ETT cuff

Attach ETT adaptor, ventilate patient, and confirm ETT position

Deflate ILMA, and remove it using the push rod, after ETT 15 mm adaptor is removed

Grasp ETT with fingers (or Magill forceps) when it is visible or palpable, continue LMA removal

Reattach adaptor to ETT, begin ventilation, and reconfirm ETT position

Secure ETT

Practicality: Reasonably expensive ($1500 for 3 adult sizes)

Portable

More complex than standard LMA: ETT insertion requires multiple attempts at times, adjustment maneuvers must be well-understood and removal of LMA without moving ETT can be awkward.

Unfamiliar to many outside of the OR environment; requires use and practice for facility

Indications: Predicted difficult airway

Difficult ventilation and/or intubation

Routine airway management for elective OR cases

Contraindications: Severe upper airway obstruction

Inaccessibility of oral cavity

Complications: Regurgitation/aspiration of gastric contents

Figure 24.3 Placement of ILMA into pharynx of cadaver specimen.

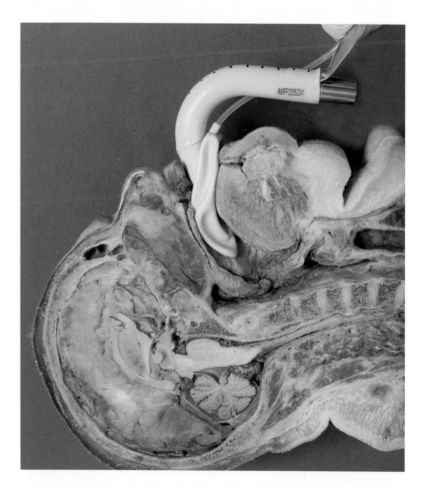

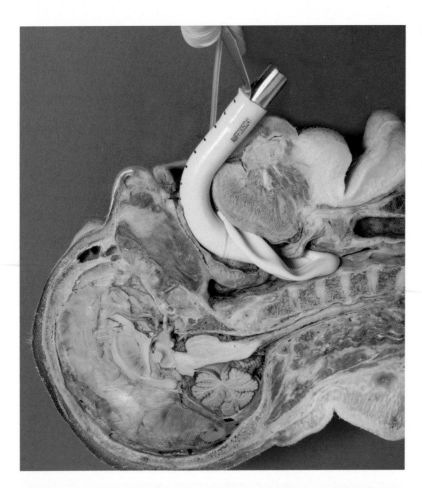

Figure 24.4 ILMA in place for ventilation.

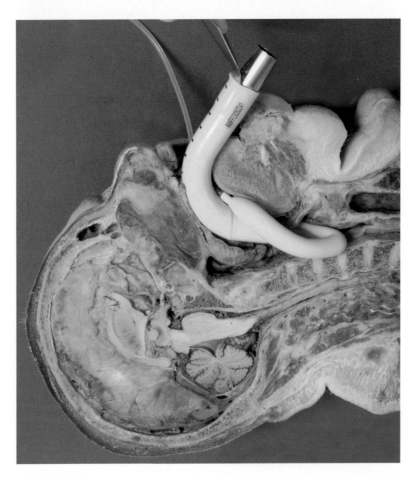

Figure 24.5 ILMA inflated to seal glottis.

Figure 24.6 ETT placed through the ILMA, entering the airway.

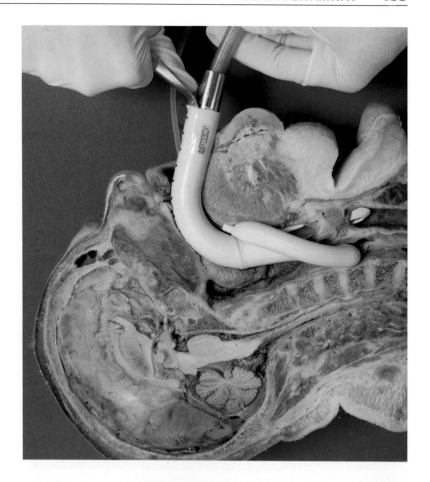

Figure 24.7 ETT passing into trachea.

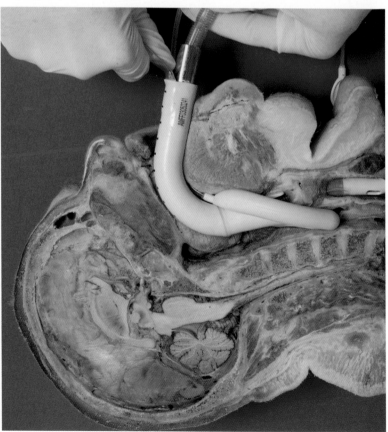

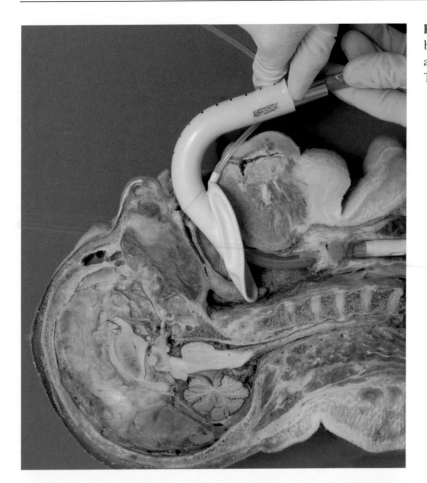

Figure 24.8 After the ETT is confirmed to be in the airway, the ILMA cuff is deflated and the ILMA device carefully removed. The ETT adaptor must be removed first.

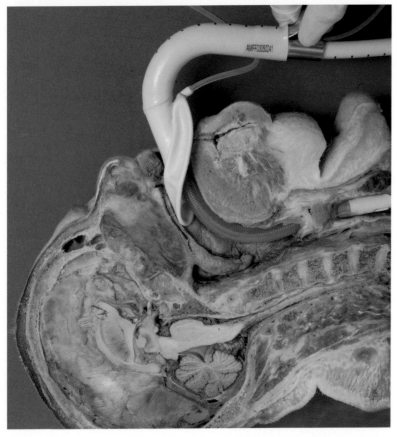

Figure 24.9 Use of push rod to stabilize ETT during LMA removal.

Figure 24.10 Grasping ETT with forceps or fingers as ILMA is extracted from mouth.

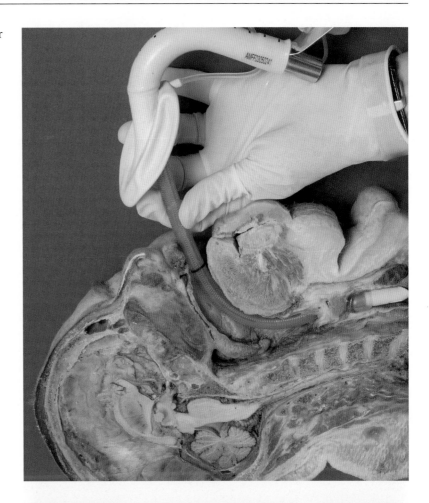

Figure 24.11 ETT now in place, ventilation is re-initiated and tube fixed.

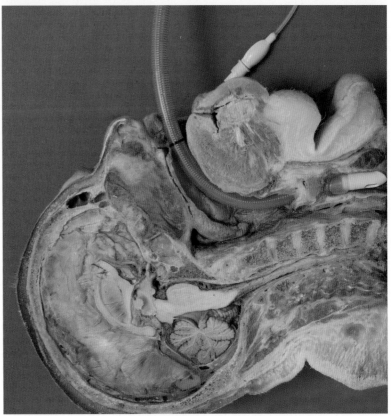

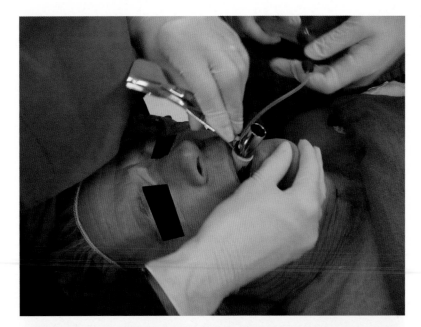

Figure 24.12 ILMA insertion.

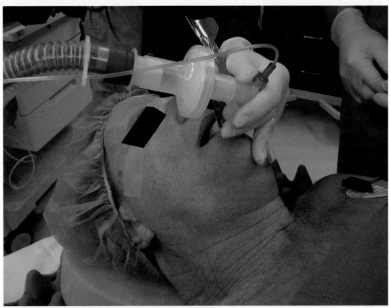

Figure 24.13 ILMA in correct position, ventilation initiated.

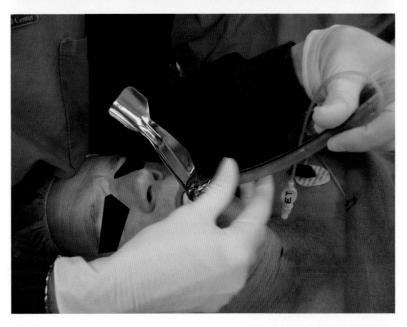

Figure 24.14 ETT insertion with black line facing cephalad. When the black band at 15 cm on the ETT reaches the lumen of the ILMA, the ETT tip is beginning to push into the pharynx, moving the epiglottic elevating bar out of the way.

Figure 24.15 Adaptor attached to ETT, ventilation confirmed.

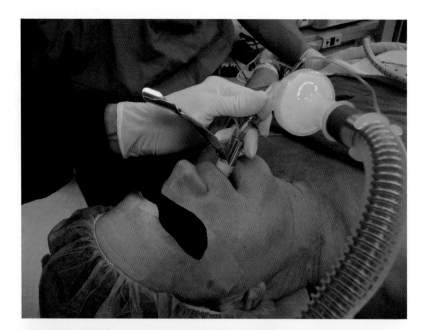

Figure 24.16 Use of push rod to remove LMA.

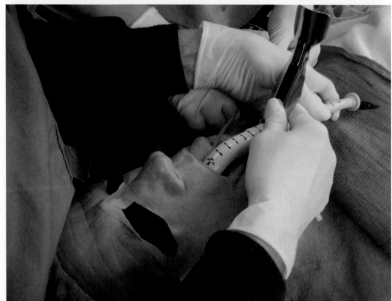

Figure 24.17 Grasping ETT with fingers to stabilize as ILMA is removed from mouth.

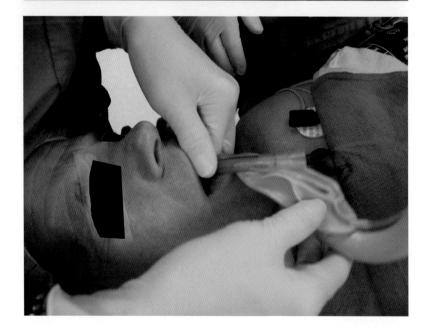

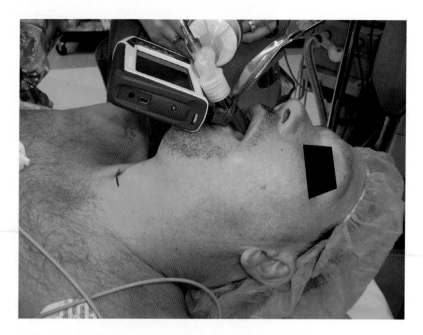

Figure 24.18 The C-Trach device: after insertion of the ILMA and ventilation confirmed, a view screen is attached.

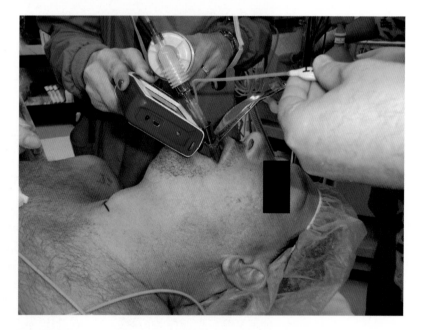

Figure 24.19 The fiberoptics in the device permit observation of ETT placement into the glottis, after which the ILMA is removed as above.

Table 24.1

Adjustment Maneuvers for Blind Intubation Through the ILMA (3)

Depth of Resistance	Likely Cause of Resistance	Corrective Action
0.0 to 1.5 cm	Epiglottic elevating bar (EEB) trapped behind cricoid cartilage	Replace ILMA with next smaller size
1.5 to 2.0 cm	Epiglottis folded down over glottic opening	Remove ETT, swing ILMA back out, up to 6.0 cm (with cuff up), replace in pharynx
2.0 to 4.0 cm	EEB lying too high	Replace ILMA with next larger size
4.0 to 6.0 cm	ETT tip wedged between mask tip and cricoid cartilage	Replace ILMA with small size

Pharyngeal trauma

Nerve injury due to prolonged compression (if LMA not removed)

Failure to seal and/or ventilate with LMA

ETT misplacement

Inability to advance ETT

REFERENCES:

1. Agro F, Brimacombe J, Carassiti M, et al. The intubating laryngeal mask. *Anesthesiology* 1998;53:1084–1090.
2. Baskett PJF, Parr MJA, Nolan JP. The intubating laryngeal mask. *Anesthesiology* 1998;53:1174–1179.
3. Brain AIJ, Verghese C, Addy EV, et al. The intubating laryngeal mask II. A preliminary clinical report of a new means of intubating the trachea. *Br J Anaesth* 1997;79:704–709.
4. Joo HS, Kapoor S, Rose DK, et al. The intubating laryngeal mask airway after induction of general anesthesia versus awake fiberoptic intubation in patients with difficult airways. *Anesth Analg* 2001;92:1342–1346.
5. Ferson DZ, Rosenblatt WH, Johansen MJ. Use of the intubating LMA-Fastrach in 254 patients with difficult-to-manage airways. *Anesthesiology* 2001;95:1175–1181.
6. Combes X, Sauvat S, Leroux B, et al. Intubating laryngeal mask airway in morbidly obese and lean patients: a comparative study. *Anesthesiology* 2005;102:1106–1109.
7. Komatsu R, Nagata O, Kamata K, et al. Comparison of the intubating laryngeal mask airway and laryngeal tube placement during manual in-line stabilization of the neck. *Anesthesia* 2005;60:113–117.
8. Wong JK, Tongier WK, Armbruster SC, et al. Use of the intubating laryngeal mask airway to facilitate awake orotracheal intubation in patients with cervical spine disorders. *J Clin Anesth* 1999;11:346–348.
9. Schuschnig C, Waltl B, Erlacher W, et al. Intubating laryngeal mask and rapid sequence induction in patients with cervical spine injury. *Anesthesia* 1999;54:793–797.
10. Asai T, Murao K, Tsutsumi T, et al. Ease of tracheal intubation through the intubating laryngeal mask airway during manual in-line head and neck stabilization. *Anesthesiology* 2000;55:82–85.
11. Rosenblatt WH, Murphy M. The intubating laryngeal mask: use of a new ventilating-intubating device in the emergency department. *Ann Emerg Med* 1999;33:234–238.

25

New Supraglottic Ventilation Devices

Concept: The success of the laryngeal mask airway (LMA) and the esophageal-tracheal combitube (ETC) in providing effective ventilation during difficult airway management has led to the release of similar devices by other manufacturers, and also spurred development of other supraglottic devices. These include the perilaryngeal airway (PLA) (Cobra PLA, Engineered Medical Systems, Indianapolis, IN) and the laryngeal tube (LT)(King LT, King Systems, Noblesville, IN) (Figs. 25.1 and 25.2). The PLA is similar in its configuration to an LMA, and is also placed in the hypopharynx, but has a larger cuff to provide an effective seal for ventilation. It is available in five sizes, including adult and pediatric. The LT is a multiuse, single lumen supraglottic ventilatory device compatible with either spontaneous ventilation (as in elective surgical cases) or positive pressure ventilation. Reminiscent of the ETC, it has an oropharyngeal and an esophageal cuff, with a ventilation aperture between the two.

Evidence: In a group of 8l patients randomized to airway management during elective surgery with either the PLA or the LMA, investigators found similar success in ventilation, but higher sealing pressures for the PLA (23 cm H_2O versus 18 cm H_2O) (1). Anecdotal reports attest to the utility of the PLA in providing ventilation in difficult airway scenarios, as well as facilitating fiberoptic bronchoscopic intubation (2,3). As with virtually all supraglottic devices, a risk of aspiration exists (4).

The LT has been shown to function well with mechanical ventilation. In 97% of 175 elective surgical cases, oxygenation, ventilation, and pulmonary mechanics were well maintained using this device (5). In a comparison of the LT with the LMA in 50 patients undergoing general anesthesia for minor surgery, the devices were equally effective in maintaining oxygenation and ventilation during controlled ventilation, with comparable insertion times (6). Mean airway leak pressures were significantly higher with the Laryngeal Tube (36 cm H_2O versus 22 cm H_2O). The LT has been utilized in difficult airway situations, including lingual tonsillar hyperplasia and morbid obesity (7), and has been effective in providing ventilation for patients undergoing cardiopulmonary resuscitation (8).

As with the LMA, high inflation pressures (greater than 60 cm H_2O) should be avoided so that pharyngeal mucosal perfusion is not compromised (9). Ideally, these cuff pressures are monitored with a manometer.

Preparation:

Same as for direct laryngoscopy (Chapter 3)
Select the appropriate size device
Lubricate the PLA or the LT
Anesthetized or unconscious, pre-oxygenated patient in neutral position (for PLA) or sniffing position (for LT)
Check the device for cuff leaks and pilot balloon integrity

Procedure for PLA insertion:

Extend the head, and ensure the cuff is completely deflated
Open the mouth
Slide the PLA into the hypopharynx until resistance is met
Pull back slightly (cuff should not be visible in mouth)
Inflate with just enough air to establish a seal
Confirm effective ventilation
Secure device to patient

Procedure for LT insertion:

Open the mouth with the nondominant hand, grasping the mandible and pulling forward
Insert the LT device, rotated 45 degrees to 90 degrees laterally, behind the tongue
Inflate cuffs of LT (one pilot balloon for both) to 60 cm H_2O pressure, or inflate to minimum volume necessary to seal the airway at the peak ventilatory pressure to be employed
Attach to breathing circuit, begin ventilation and slowly withdraw the airway until ventilation is optimal
Confirm effective ventilation
Readjust cuff inflation to 60 cm H_2O (or to volume that just seals)
Secure device to patient

Figure 25.1 Cobra Peri-Laryngeal Airway. (Courtesy of Engineered Medical Systems, Indianapolis, IN.) Note two devices are pictured.

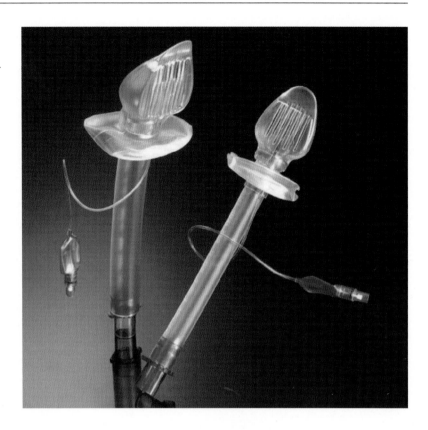

Figure 25.2 King Laryngeal Tube in three sizes. (Courtesy of King Medical Systems, Noblesville, IN.)

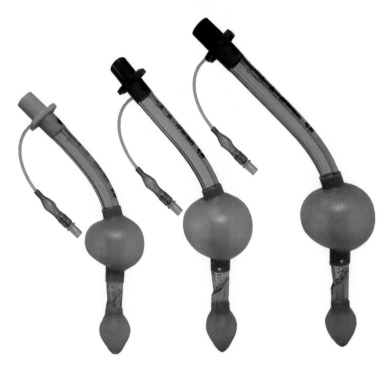

Practicality: Portable
Inexpensive
Both devices will likely be unfamiliar to those outside the OR and will require practice on mannequins or normal patients for facility in their use

Indications: Elective airway during surgery
Emergency ventilation when face mask ventilation fails

Contraindications: Inaccessibility of the oral cavity
Full stomach or aspiration risk (except in emergencies)
Severe supraglottic obstruction

Complications: Inability to ventilate
Potential pharyngeal or esophageal trauma from insertion
Regurgitation and aspiration of gastric contents
Overinflation of cuffs, with resultant pharyngeal mucosal injury

REFERENCES:

1. Akca O, Wadwha A, Sengupta P, et al. The new perilaryngeal airway (Cobra PLA) is as efficient as the Laryngeal Mask Airway (LMA) but provides better airway sealing pressures. *Anesth Analg* 2004;99:272–278.
2. Szmuk P, Ezri T, Akca O, et al. Use of a new supraglottic airway device-the Cobra PLA-in a "difficult to intubate/difficult to ventilate" scenario. *Acta Anaesth Scand* 2005,49:421–423.
3. Szmuk P. Cobra PLA as a conduit for flexible bronchoscopy in a child under general anesthesia. *Br J Anaesth* 2005;94:548–549.
4. Cook TM, Lowe JM. An evaluation of the Cobra Perilaryngeal Airway: study halted after two cases of pulmonary aspiration. *Anesthesia* 2005;60:791.
5. Gaitini LA, Vaida SJ, Somri M, et al. An evaluation of the Laryngeal Tube during general anesthesia using mechanical ventilation. *Anesth Analg* 2003;96:1750–1755.
6. Ocker H, Wenzel V, Schumucker P, et al. A comparison of the Laryngeal Tube with the Laryngeal Mask Airway during routine surgical procedures. *Anesth Analg* 2002;95:1094–1097.
7. Matioc AA, Olson J. Use of the Laryngeal Tube TM in two unexpected difficult airway situations: lingual tonsillar hyperplasia and morbid obesity. *Can J Anaesth* 2004;51:1018–1021.
8. Asai T, Shingu K. The laryngeal tube. *Br J Anaesth* 2005;95: 729–736.
9. Matioc AA, Arndt G. The laryngeal tube and pharyngeal mucosal pressure. *Can J Anaesth* 2003;50:525–526.

26

Transtracheal "Jet" Ventilation

Concept: At times, supraglottic ventilation devices, such as the esophageal-tracheal combitube (ETC) and the laryngeal mask airway (LMA), are rendered ineffectual as emergency ventilation devices by supraglottic swelling or glottic pathology, such as abscess, tumor or foreign body, or by unfavorable anatomy that precludes their placement, such as limited mouth opening. Under such circumstances, an approach to emergent ventilation that utilizes an infra-glottic, percutaneous route is an alternative. Transtracheal "jet" ventilation (TTJV) requires the placement of a large bore catheter through the cricothyroid membrane, or even directly into the trachea (1,2). This is connected to a high-pressure oxygen source, preferably by a tight-fitting Luer-lock connection. The delivery of oxygen through this apparatus can be used to both oxygenate and ventilate the patient through the catheter inserted into the airway (3–5). Connecting the catheter to a resuscitation bag or anesthesia circuit using the adaptor from a size 3.0 ETT along with a 3 mL syringe is far less effective in delivering adequate tidal volumes with this technique (6). A 50 pounds per square inch (psi) oxygen source is preferred, via either an oxygen cylinder with a two-stage regulator, or the hospital wall oxygen system (1,7). A variety of components can be assembled piecemeal to create a useable delivery system, but commercially available systems are more reliable and are reasonably priced (1,8). Reinforced catheters are available from a variety of manufacturers, to reduce the likelihood of kinking after insertion into the airway.

When oxygen at high pressure (20 psi to 50 psi) and high flow (0.5 liter/sec to 1.0 liter/sec) is delivered by TTJV, air may be entrained at the catheter tip, augmenting the tidal volume and increasing the risk of barotrauma. Given the flow rates and pressures involved, adequate tidal volume for an adult usually can be delivered in 0.5 second to 1.0 second. Utilizing a lung model with a set compliance of 50 mL/cm H_2O, a 1 second inspiratory time and a 50 psi oxygen source, tidal volumes generated vary from about 600 mL with an 18-gauge catheter to over 1,200 mL with a 14-gauge catheter (1).

Evidence: TTJV was demonstrated to provide adequate ventilation in cardiac arrest patients as early as 1972, when Jacobs described its use in 40 cases (5). While utilizing a high-pressure oxygen source, the author was able to maintain an average PaO_2 of 300 mm Hg, and a $PaCO_2$ of 22 mm Hg with peak airway pressures of 15 cm to 25 cm H_2O. In 1975, Smith described the use of TTJV in 80 patients who underwent airway surgery under general anesthesia (9). Fifty-two of these cases involved elective use of the technique, while 28 of the patients were managed while in respiratory distress. Provided that adequate pressures are utilized to provide necessary flow rates, several investigators have demonstrated that normocarbia can be maintained while ventilating patients with TTJV (4,5). Many of the patients described in these investigations were under general anesthesia, in contrast to patients in acute respiratory failure who are frequently encountered in the hospital wards, intensive care units, or emergency department. TTJV also has been useful in high-grade upper airway obstruction, as in the case of a patient with a large carcinoma at the base of the tongue who sustained a respiratory arrest (10). TTJV has been used effectively as a ventilation strategy in cannot-intubate, cannot-ventilate (failed airway) situations (1,7,8). The technique has also proven useful in pediatric airway emergencies (11).

Preparation for TTJV using a commercially available device (Figs. 26.1 and 26.2):

Preparation for direct laryngoscopy (see Chapter 3)
Anesthetized or unconscious, pre-oxygenated patient with head extension to allow access to cricothyroid membrane
Fill 10-mL syringe halfway with saline, attach to 16-gauge or 14-gauge 2-inch intravenous catheter-needle (or to a catheter manufactured for this purpose)
Attach the high-pressure tubing of the device to 50 psi wall oxygen source (or oxygen tank with two stage regulator)
Check integrity of components, test oxygen flow
Prepare the neck over the cricothyroid membrane with antiseptic solution, if time allows

Procedure (Figs. 26.3 to 26.10):

With nondominant hand, grasp thyroid cartilage using thumb and long finger, and palpate cricothyroid membrane with index finger
Puncture the cricothyroid membrane, with needle at 30-degree angle to skin

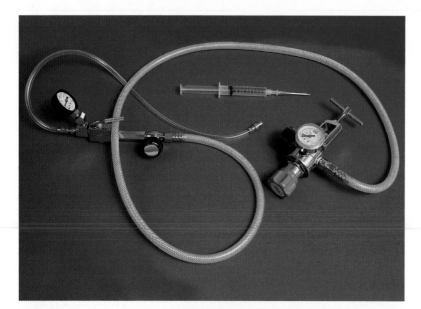

Figure 26.1 Commercially available TTJV apparatus.

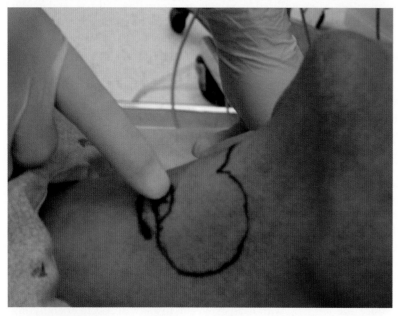

Figure 26.2 Palpating the cricothyroid membrane between the marked thyroid and cricoid cartilages.

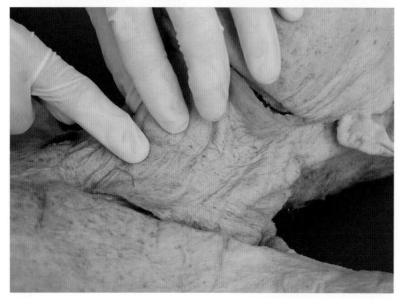

Figure 26.3 Cricothyroid membrane demonstrated in cadaver specimen.

Figure 26.4 Puncture of cricothyroid membrane.

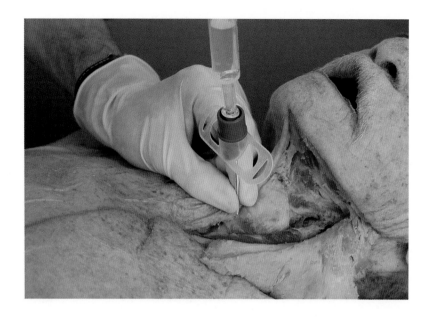

Figure 26.5 Advancing the catheter caudad into the trachea.

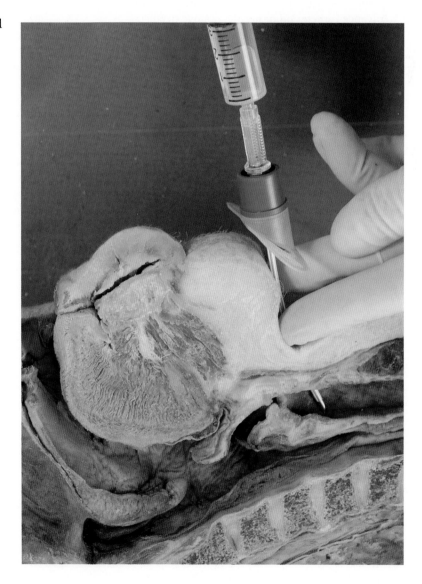

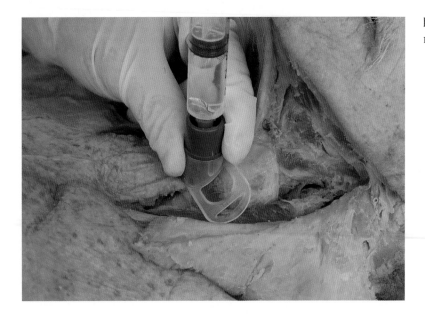

Figure 26.6 Catheter now seated in airway, needle has been removed.

Ensure tracheal entry: withdraw air into syringe

Advance catheter off of needle, remove needle

ASSISTANT is assigned to HOLD catheter hub AT ALL TIMES

Confirm tracheal position of catheter by free withdrawal of air from catheter with syringe

Attach high pressure oxygen source with Luer-lock to catheter

Begin TTJV, at the lowest possible pressure (20 cm to 30 cm H_2O), observing for chest rise and breath sounds

For small children (younger than 5 years of age), a self-inflating bag with oxygen may be used, rather than high-pressure oxygen, to reduce the likelihood of barotrauma (an adaptor from a size 3 ETT fits to the catheter in the CTM, allowing the bag to be attached), but ventilation is less effective than with a high-pressure oxygen delivery system

Cease inspiratory airflow as soon as chest rise noted

Ensure adequate airflow out of trachea with oral and/or nasal airways and jaw thrust

Conduct inspiration/exhalation at 1:3 or 1:4 ratio, to allow adequate time for passive exhalation and avoidance of barotrauma

Begin search for definitive airway —fiberoptic bronchoscope (FOB), retrograde, cricothyrotomy, and optical stylet are all possibilities—direct laryngoscopy may also be facilitated by high pressure gas exiting the larynx, making its location more obvious

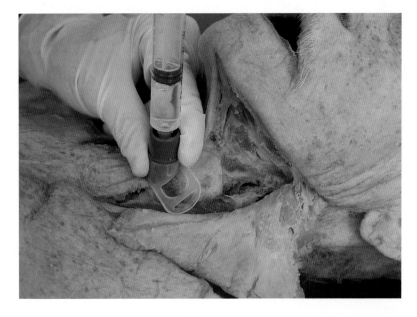

Figure 26.7 Attach syringe to catheter, pull back bubbles to reconfirm position in airway.

Figure 26.8 An assistant should now be designated to hold the hub of the catheter until a definitive airway is established.

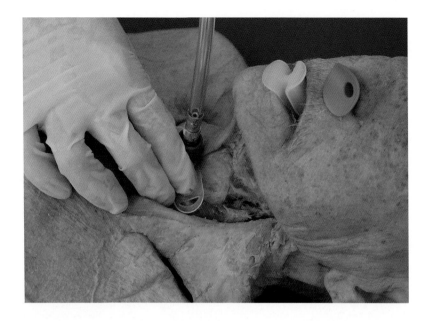

Figure 26.9 Attach TTJV system with Luer-lock, begin ventilation. Oral and nasal airways should be in place to ensure exhalation is unimpeded, or barotrauma may occur.

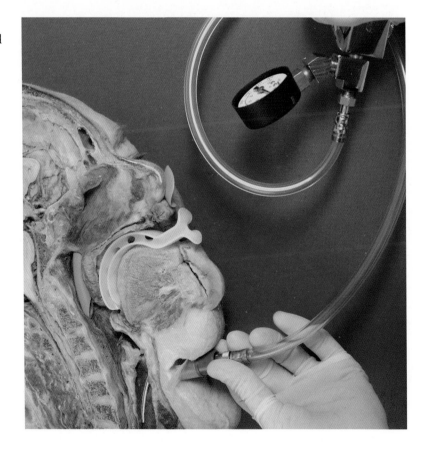

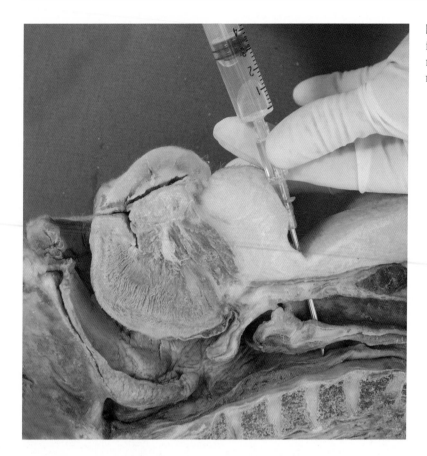

Figure 26.10 If the needle is advanced too far during puncture of the cricothyroid membrane, perforation of the esophagus may occur.

Practicality: Reasonably inexpensive: ($200 to $300 for available system)

Commercial systems are portable and simple

Unfamiliar: user should practice hooking up components, and identifying and instrumenting cricothyroid membrane

Indications: Failed intubation and/or failed ventilation

Inaccessibility to oral cavity in patient requiring emergent ventilation

Severe facial trauma with inaccessible airway

Severe upper airway obstruction precluding other, supraglottic, emergent ventilation techniques, or failure of these techniques

Contraindications: Bleeding diathesis (relative)

Complete upper airway obstruction (predisposes to severe barotrauma)

Inability to palpate cricothyroid membrane

Complications: Laryngeal or tracheal trauma from needle stick

Esophageal perforation or entry with needle

Failure to ventilate or oxygenate due to misplaced or kinked catheter

Subcutaneous air insufflation due to misplaced needle

Bleeding or hematoma

Barotrauma: mediastinal air, pneumopericardium, pneumothorax, tension pneumothorax

"Stacking" of breaths due to inadequate expiratory time, with increased intrathoracic pressure, reduced cardiac preload and hypotension

REFERENCES:

1. Benumof JL, Scheller MS. The importance of transtracheal jet ventilation in the management of the difficult airway. *Anesthesiology* 1989;71:769–778.
2. Jacobs HB, Smyth NPD, Witorsch P. Transtracheal catheter ventilation. *Chest* 1974;65:36–40.
3. Klain M, Smith RB. High frequency percutaneous transtracheal ventilation. *Crit Care Med* 1977;5:280–287.
4. Weymuller EA, Paugh D, Pavlin EG, et al. Management of difficult airway problems with percutaneous transtracheal jet ventilation. *Ann Otol Rhinol Laryngol* 1987;96:34–37.

5. Jacobs HB. Needle catheter brings oxygen to the trachea. *JAMA* 1972;222:1231–1233.

6. Dunlap LB. A modified, simple device for the emergency administration of percutaneous transtracheal jet ventilation. *J Am Coll Emerg Phys* 1978;7:42–46.

7. Delisser EA, Muravchick S. Emergency transtracheal ventilation. *Anesthesiology* 1981;55:606–607.

8. Scuderi PE, McLeskey CH, Comer PB. Emergency percutaneous transtracheal ventilation during anesthesia using readily available equipment. *Anesth Analg* 1982;61:867–870.

9. Smith RB, Schaer WB, Pfaeffle H. Percutaneous transtracheal ventilation for anesthesia. *Can J Anaesth* 1975;22:607–609.

10. Biro P, Moe KS. Emergency transtracheal jet ventilation in highgrade airway obstruction. *J Clin Anaesth* 1975;22:604–606.

11. Ravussin P, Bayer-Berger M, Monnier P, et al. Percutaneous transtracheal ventilation for laser endoscopic procedures in infants and small children with laryngeal obstruction. *Can J Anaesth* 1987;34:83–86.

Intubation through Laryngeal Mask Airway or Intubation Laryngeal Mask Airway with a Bougie, Lighted Stylet, or Optical Stylet

Concept: As noted in previous chapters, both the laryngeal mask airway (LMA) and the intubating laryngeal mask airway (ILMA) are optimally positioned when lying in the hypopharynx, with the mask atop the glottic opening. This position facilitates passage of a guiding catheter through the tube of the device, often directly into the glottis. An endotracheal tube (ETT) can then be passed over it and into the trachea. The LMA lumen limits the size of the ETT to be passed to a size 6.0-mm internal diameter (ID) in a size 3 or 4 LMA, or a 7.0-mm ID in a size 5 LMA. The 6.0 ETT can project only a short distance past the mask of the LMA, into the larynx, due to the length of these tubes when compared with the length of the LMA itself. In contrast, the ILMA device, in all three sizes, has a lumen large enough to accommodate size 8.0 ETTs. Further, the design of the ILMA and the push rod included with it facilitate removal of the device after the ETT is seated and confirmed to be in the airway.

Evidence: Anecdotal reports exist that describe the placement of a bougie through an LMA to improve the potential for accurate intubation (1). However, this technique is probably no better than simply inserting an ETT through the LMA, without guidance (2), which has a high failure rate (3). These blind techniques are less successful than those which allow visualization of the airway. In a comparison of intubation through the LMA with the use of a bougie, versus the ILMA combined with the use of a fiberscope for direct visualization, in patients with in-line cervical immobilization, Asai reported a success rate of 85% for the latter combination, but less than 50% for the former (4).

A technique that has generated more interest, and is likely to improve accuracy of ETT placement, is use of a lightwand, placed through a LMA or ILMA device, to allow the practitioner to guide an ETT into the larynx with transillumination. Agro et al made use of this technique in 114 patients under anesthesia, after LMA insertion. After successful LMA placement, the lightwand and ETT were inserted into the LMA, projecting 1.5 cm beyond the grill (5). In 78% of patients, the authors were able to intubate

without repositioning the LMA, while 10% required repositioning, and 9% required a change to different size LMA. Three patients were impossible to intubate in this manner.

Nijima et al reported use of the Trachlite (Laerdahl, Long Beach, CA) lightwand with the intubating LMA (6). In their approach, the stiff internal stylet of the lightwand is withdrawn, and the device is threaded through the Murphy eye of the ETT, then its tip placed through the ILMA lumen. With gentle insertion of the lightwand, probing for the glottis, transillumination was used to guide the ETT into the larynx. Dimitriou et al evaluated the ILMA as an effective intubating device utilizing a flexible lightwand in unexpected failed laryngoscopy in 11,621 patients. The study participants could not intubate a total of 44 patients with direct laryngoscopy in three attempts (7). Ventilation with the ILMA was accomplished in all of these 44 patients; lightwand-guided intubation through the ILMA was successful in 86% on the first attempt, 12% on one or more subsequent attempts, and failed in one patient (2%). An optical stylet has also been utilized for intubation through the ILMA (8).

Preparation for lightwand-assisted intubation through the LMA:

>   Same as for LMA insertion (see Chapter 23)
>   Lubricate lightwand and ETT
>   Place lightwand through ETT, with tip flush with end of tube
>   Anesthetized or unconscious, pre-oxygenated patient in neutral position

Procedure for lightwand-guided intubation through LMA (Figs. 27.1 to 27.3):

>   Insert LMA (see Chapter 23)
>   Establish optimal ventilation pattern
>   Insert lightwand/ETT through lumen of LMA, to project 1.5 cm from the grill of the distal LMA lumen
>   Alternatively, insert ILMA and establish optimal ventilation, then place ETT/lightwand through lumen
>   Observe neck for transillumination

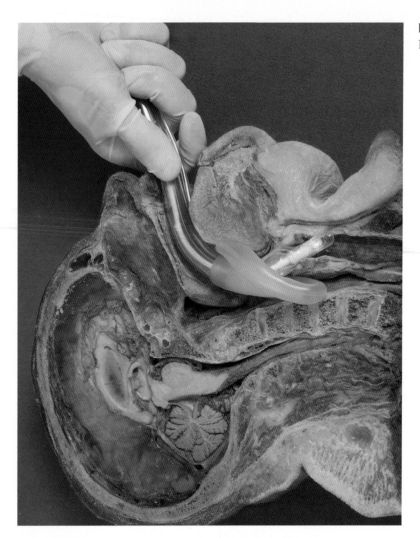

Figure 27.1 Insertion of ETT/lightwand into LMA situated in cadaver specimen.

Advance lightwand when transillumination indicates glottic entry

If halo of light not seen over the crycothyroid membrane (CTM), the LMA should be repositioned, depending on the location of visible light, by advancing, withdrawing, or rotating it, or by placing a different size LMA (or ILMA)

Advance lightwand/ETT until halo passes beyond CTM to suprasternal notch

Advance ETT and remove lightwand

Ventilate through ETT, confirm placement in airway

Leave LMA device in place with deflated cuff (or, if using ILMA, remove it with push rod)

Fix ETT/LMA in place

Practicality: Simple, portable, affordable
    Unfamiliar: requires practice to fit lightwand/LMA through device, and familiarity with transillumination of the larynx

Indications: Inability to intubate trachea by direct laryngoscopy
    Copious blood or secretions in airway (precluding techniques that require glottic visualization)
    Necessity of ETT after emergency ventilation with LMA

Contraindications: Laryngeal fracture or trauma
    Inability to ventilate through LMA
    Upper airway obstruction

Complications: ETT misplacement in esophagus
    Inability to advance lightwand/ETT
    Laryngeal or pharyngeal trauma from blind probing

Figure 27.2 Lightwand/ETT advanced into airway. Note that only a few centimeters of the 6.0 cm ETT enters the larynx when inserted through the LMA.

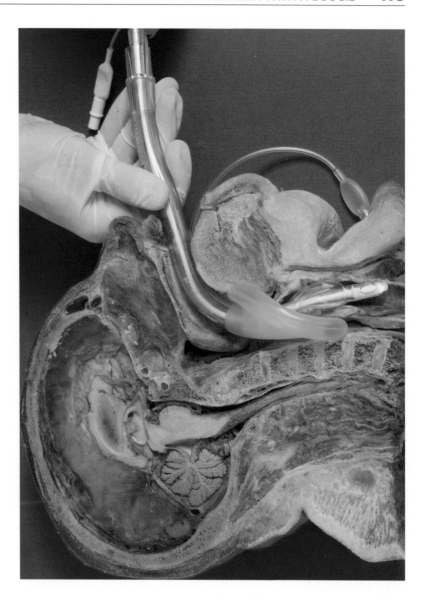

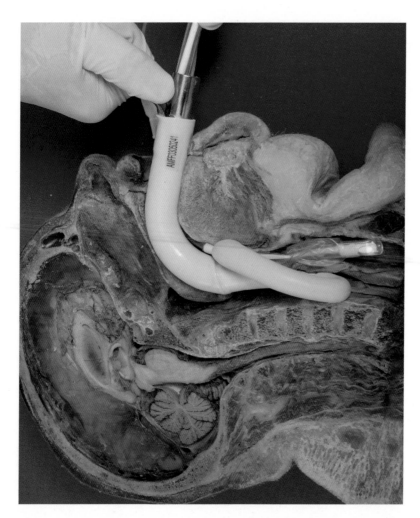

Figure 27.3 A larger ETT may be inserted, and to a greater depth in the larynx, when the ILMA is used with the lightwand.

REFERENCES:

1. Murdoch JAC. Emergency tracheal intubation using a gum bougie through a laryngeal mask airway. *Anesthesia* 2005;60:626–627.
2. Ahmed AB, Nathanson MH, Gajraj NM. Tracheal intubation through the laryngeal mask airway using a gum elastic bougie: the effect of head position. *J Clin Anesth* 2001;13:427–429.
3. Benumof JL. Laryngeal mask airway and the ASA difficult airway algorithm. *Anesthesiology* 1996;84:686–699.
4. Asai T, Murao K, Tsutsumi T, et al. Ease of tracheal intubation through the intubating laryngeal mask during manual in-line head and neck stabilization. *Anesthesiology* 2000;55:82–85.
5. Agro F, Brimacombe J, Carassiti M, et al. Use of a lighted stylet for intubation via the laryngeal mask airway. *Can J Anaesth* 1998;45:556–560.
6. Niijima K, Seto A, Aoyama K, et al. An illuminating stylet as an aid for tracheal intubation via the intubating laryngeal mask airway. *Anesth Analg* 1999;88:470–471.
7. Dimitriou V, Voyagis GS, Brimacombe JR. Flexible lightwand-guided tracheal intubation with the intubating laryngeal mask Fastrach in adults after unpredicted laryngoscope-guided tracheal intubation. *Anesthesiology* 2002;96: 296–299.
8. Agro FE, Antonelli S, Cataldo R. Use of Shikani flexible seeing stylet for intubation via the intubating laryngeal mask airway. *Can J Anaesth* 2005;52:657–658.

28

Retrograde Intubation and Flexible Fiberoptic Bronchoscope Intubation

Concept: Retrograde intubation (RI) was discussed in Chapter 18. While reported success rates are high, RI remains a "blind" procedure: the endotracheal tube (ETT) is advanced with wire guidance, and there is no visualization of the glottis as the tube is moved forward. The ETT may move out of the larynx, into the esophagus, or kink, with failure to advance, after the wire and guide catheters are removed. To improve the success of RI, it can be combined with a fiberoptic bronchoscope (FOB) in order to obtain direct visualization of the airway as the tube is advanced, and immediately confirm appropriate placement of the ETT (1,2). When the guidewire is retrieved from the mouth, it is fed through the working channel of the FOB from distal to proximal. The FOB is then fed over the wire to the glottis. After the wire is removed, the FOB acts as a visualizing guide catheter. This reduces the chance that the ETT will be dislodged from the trachea during the blind technique, as the glottis can be visualized throughout.

Evidence: Case reports attest to the utility of this combination of airway management techniques (1–3).

Preparation:

  Same as for retrograde intubation (see Chapter 19)
  Same as for fiberoptic bronchoscopy, except that this combination would most likely be used in an unconscious patient, so that topicalization is unlikely to be necessary (see Chapter 20)
  Remove the rubber or plastic cover from the suction port of the FOB, to allow wire to emerge from the suction channel

Procedure (Figs. 28.1 to 28.5):

  Carry out RI steps 1 through 5. No guide catheter is used
  Retrieve wire from mouth, thread into suction channel at tip of the FOB, until it emerges from suction port

Pull end of wire out of proximal end of FOB, clamping it or having assistant hold it throughout the ETT insertion
Maintain tension on wire, and insert FOB along it (using wire as a guide to FOB advancement)
Jaw thrust and/or direct laryngoscopy will likely be required
Visualize larynx, advance FOB through it, to point of wire entry into larynx
Advance FOB into trachea, if possible (if FOB will not advance past glottis due to wire, wire can be cut and removed to allow scope to pass)
Carefully remove guidewire without dislodging FOB from larynx
Advance FOB to within sight of carina
Slide ETT over FOB, confirm position, remove FOB
Fix ETT in place

Practicality: Complex, unfamiliar: requires practice
Expensive due to use of FOB
Not easily portable, due to FOB
All of the logistics issues of FOB apply (see Chapter 20)

Indications: Difficult Airway Predicted
Inability to intubate, with preserved ability to ventilate

Contraindications: Copious secretions/blood in airway
Inability to ventilate, due to time required for this procedure
Distorted, traumatized, or unrecognizable laryngeal anatomy

Complications: Complications of both retrograde intubation and FOB intubation are possible with this combined technique (see Chapters 19 and 20)

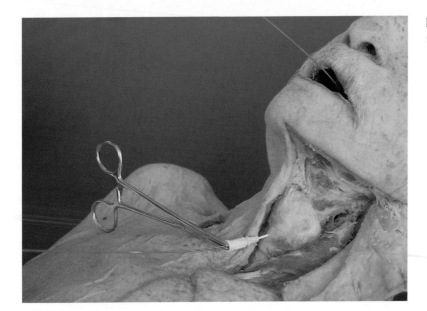

Figure 28.1 Wire has been retrieved from the mouth during RI in cadaver specimen.

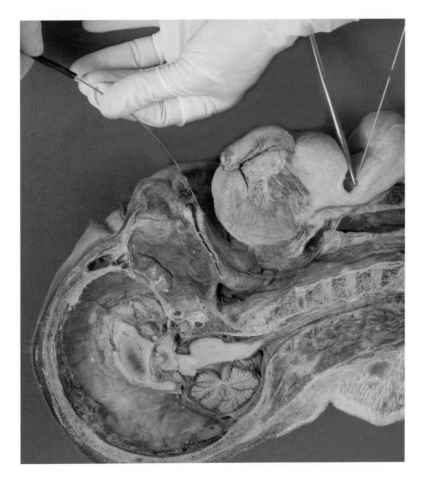

Figure 28.2 RI wire is now inserted into suction channel of FOB.

Figure 28.3 FOB is advanced over the wire, while maintaining tension on wire.

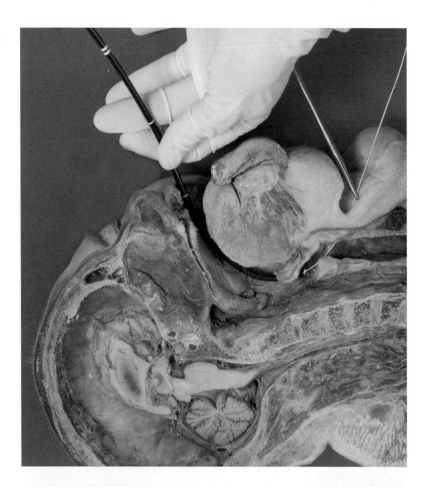

Figure 28.4 When the tip of the FOB abuts the CTM, the wire is removed, from either the CTM or the suction port of the scope.

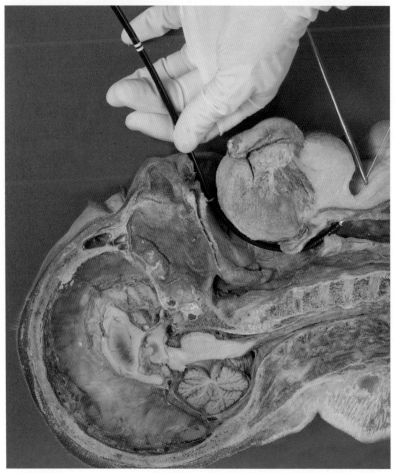

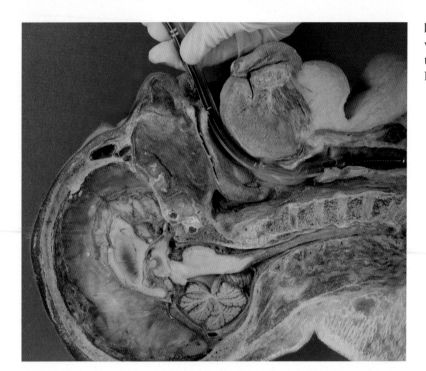

Figure 28.5 After the wire is removed, advance the FOB distally in the trachea until the carina is visualized. Then advance the ETT as in any FOB-guided intubation.

REFERENCES:

1. Lechmann MJ, Donahoo JS, Macvaugh H. Endotracheal intubation using percutaneous retrograde guidewire insertion followed by antegrade fiberoptic bronchoscopy. *Crit Care Med* 1986;14:589–590.

2. Finucane BT, Santora AH. *Principles of airway management,* 2nd ed. St. Louis: Mosby; 1996: 69–107.
3. Tobias R. Increased success with retrograde guide for endotracheal intubation. *Anesth Analg* 1983;62:366–367.

29

Flexible Fiberoptic Bronchoscope Intubation through the Laryngeal Mask Airway

Concept: One aspect of intubation with a fiberoptic bronchoscope (FOB) that can be frustrating is the tendency to advance the scope into the pharynx off of the midline, failing to view the glottis and becoming "lost" in the pharyngeal mucosa. The laryngeal mask airway (LMA) provides an excellent introducer for the FOB, since it is usually positioned directly atop the glottis, and whether the epiglottis is held open or folded down, it facilitates passage of the tip of the scope into the airway (1). The size 4 LMA, in both reusable and disposable versions, can only admit a size 6.0-mm internal diameter (ID) or (at best) size 6.5-mm ID. While such a tube is adequate in diameter for ventilation of most adults, its length is foreshortened compared with larger diameter ETTs, and it reaches only about 1 cm to 2 cm past the vocal cords and into the larynx when passed through the LMA device. Therefore, long-term stability of this ETT may be an issue, as even minor movement of the head or neck may dislodge it. Furthermore, it is difficult to remove the LMA without dislodging the ETT. However, for short-term use, as in the operating room (OR), or for emergency ventilation followed by intubation during difficult airway management in other settings, the use of the LMA to assist with FOB intubation is a valuable technique.

Evidence: A number of case reports support the value of using FOB to intubate through the LMA (1–4).

Preparation:

Prepare for LMA insertion (see Chapter 23)
Prepare for FOB intubation, using a 4 mm scope (larger scopes will be difficult to insert through the 6.0-mm ID or 6.5-mm ID ETT) (see Chapter 20)
If difficult ventilation requires emergent LMA insertion, then the ETT/FOB can be inserted through it during ongoing ventilation, utilizing an FOB adaptor in the circuit: the tight fit of the ETT in LMA lumen allows ventilation through the ETT during insertion

Anesthetized, pre-oxygenated patient in neutral or sniffing position

Procedure (Figs. 29.1 to 29.6):

Insert LMA (see Chapter 23)
Confirm adequate ventilation through LMA
After FOB is prepared, insert its tip into the proximal end of the LMA
An FOB elbow adaptor can be attached to the 15 mm adaptor of the ETT, and the ETT advanced through the LMA to its grill; attaching a breathing circuit to the FOB adaptor will then allow ongoing ventilation during FOB intubation attempts
Advance FOB through LMA, and visualize glottis beyond the grill at the end of the LMA lumen
Push scope tip through LMA grill, enter glottis, and advance until carina is visualized
Advance ETT over FOB until its adaptor is flush against the adaptor of the LMA
Remove FOB
Confirm breath sounds, ETCO$_2$, and tube position
Deflate cuff of LMA, but do not attempt to remove
Secure ETT/LMA in place
If long-term intubation is required, efforts should be made to place a longer ETT into the trachea for improved airway security (using FOB or tube changer device)

Practicality: Expensive due to incorporation of FOB
Neither simple nor familiar: requires training and practice
Portability compromised due to FOB
All of the logistics issues of FOB apply (see Chapter 20)

Indications: Difficult ventilation (LMA utilized initially as a lifesaving ventilation technique, followed by FOB intubation)
Difficult intubation (LMA utilized as a guidance device for FOB)

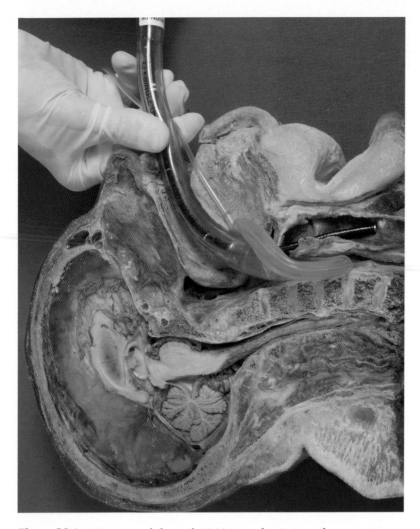

Figure 29.1 FOB inserted through LMA into glottis, in cadaver specimen.

Figure 29.2 ETT is pushed through the mask of the LMA, into the larynx. Because of its relatively short length, the 6.0 ETT protrudes only a limited distance into the larynx.

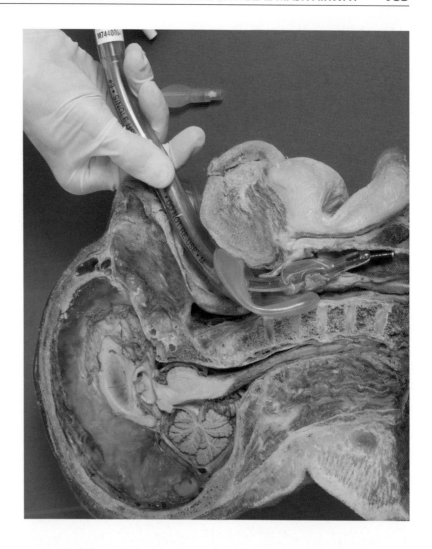

Figure 29.3 FOB insertion into LMA after ventilation optimized.

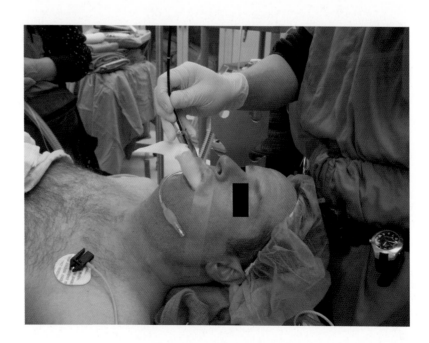

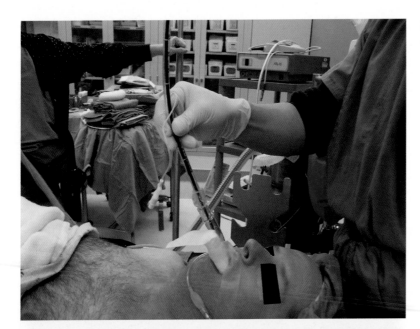

Figure 29.4 Introduction of the 6.0 ETT into the LMA.

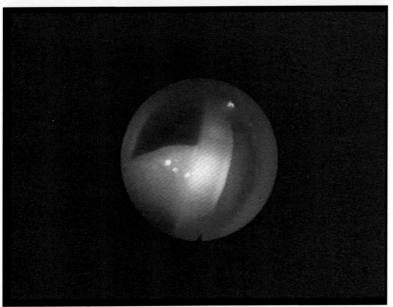

Figure 29.5 FOB image from inside the LMA reveals the epiglottis, just beyond the grill which marks the end of the LMA lumen.

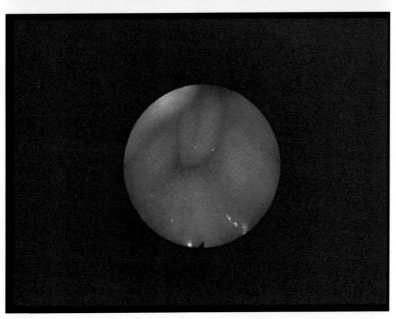

Figure 29.6 When the tip of the FOB is advanced through the grill of the LMA, the glottis is usually readily apparent.

Contraindications: Copious blood or secretions in
airway
Inaccessibility of oral cavity
(unable to insert LMA)
Severe upper airway obstruction

Complications: Complications of both LMA insertion
and FOB intubation are possible
with this combination technique
(see Chapters 20 and 23)

REFERENCES:

1. Benumof JL. Use of the laryngeal mask airway to facilitate fiberoptic bronchoscopic intubation. *Anesth Analg* 1992;74:313–315.
2. Benumof JL. Laryngeal mask airway and the ASA difficult airway algorithm. *Anesthesiology* 1996;84:686–699.
3. Heath ML, Allagain J. Intubation through the laryngeal mask. *Anesthesiology* 1991;76:545–548.
4. Orebaugh SL. Airway obstruction secondary to prolonged shoulder arthroscopy. *Anesthesiology* 2003;99:1456–1458.

30

Flexible Fiberoptic Bronchosope Intubation through the Intubating Laryngeal Mask Airway

Concept: Just as the laryngeal mask airway (LMA) does, the intubating laryngeal mask airway (ILMA) provides an excellent conduit from the mouth to the laryngeal orifice, sitting astride the glottis when properly placed. Some differences between these two ventilation adjuncts exist: the steel barrel of the ILMA makes a right angle as it enters the pharynx, as opposed to the gradual curve of the standard LMA lumen; the distal end of the ILMA lumen is guarded by an epiglottic elevating bar, rather than a grid; and the barrel of the ILMA is larger than that of the standard LMA, as it was designed to facilitate intubation of the trachea. The size 3, 4, and 5 ILMA all permit intubation with an 8.0 internal diameter ETT. The provider may insert an ILMA and immediately choose a fiberoptic bronchoscope (FOB) for guided intubation, or may choose to attempt blind intubation through the device and call the FOB into play only if this fails.

Evidence: The utility of intubation through the ILMA using FOB guidance has been established through several case series and comparative trials. Joo randomized 38 patients with known difficult airways to either awake intubation with FOB or to intubation after anesthesia with ILMA (1). In half of the latter group, the patients could not be intubated blindly with ILMA. However, in all of these, FOB was used successfully to intubate through the device. Ferson investigated the utility of ILMA in patients with known or suspected difficult airways (cervical immobilization; failed intubation during direct laryngoscopy; or distorted airway anatomy due to tumor, surgery, or radiation therapy) (2). In 54 of 254 patients, FOB was chosen to guide intubation through the ILMA device from the outset, while in the other 200, blind intubation was initiated (up to five attempts). The FOB was successful in 100% of the designated cases, on the first attempt. In seven cases selected for blind intubation, the ETT could not be placed in the trachea, and FOB was utilized for rescue, which was also successful on the first attempt in all cases.

Preparation:

Same as for ILMA (see Chapter 24)
Same as for FOB (see Chapter 20)
Slip ETT over FOB, after lubrication

Patient should be anesthetized, pre-oxygenated, in neutral or sniffing position; the procedure may also be conducted in the awake patient with topical anesthesia or nerve blocks to anesthetize the oropharyngeal and laryngeal mucosa

Procedure (Figs. 30.1 to 30.8):

Insert ILMA (see Chapter 24)
Confirm optimum position and ventilation through the ILMA
Place ETT through ILMA lumen to the 15 cm band (black band around ETT). The tip of the ETT is now lifting the epiglottic elevating bar, facilitating FOB passage into glottis
Alternatively, place the FOB tip through the ILMA, past the epiglottic elevating bar, into airway, then advance the ETT
An FOB elbow adaptor may be attached to the 15 mm ETT adaptor, and a breathing circuit likewise attached, to allow ongoing ventilation through the ETT/LMA during intubation attempts
Visualize glottis, enter larynx and trachea with tip of FOB
Advance the ETT, confirming correct placement with direct visualization through FOB
Ventilate through ETT for further confirmation
Remove ILMA device (see Chapter 24)
Attach circuit to ETT, re-confirm placement with breath sounds, chest rise, and $ETCO_2$
Secure ETT

Practicality: Complex and unfamiliar: requires practice in vitro and in vivo
Expensive (both devices)
Portability and logistic support are issues with FOB (see Chapter 20)

Indications: Failed intubation with blind ILMA attempts
Failed intubation with direct laryngoscopy
Failed ventilation (ILMA quickly inserted as rescue device, followed by FOB intubation with ongoing ventilation)

Figure 30.1 ILMA in appropriate position in cadaver specimen.

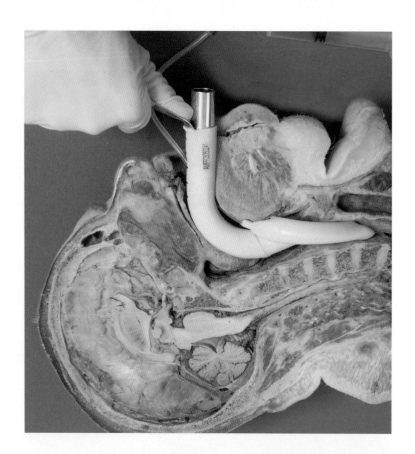

Figure 30.2 ILMA with FOB placed through it.

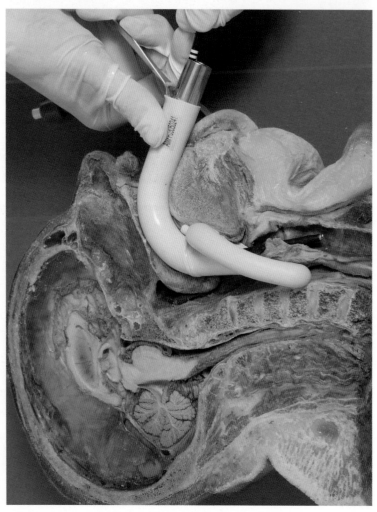

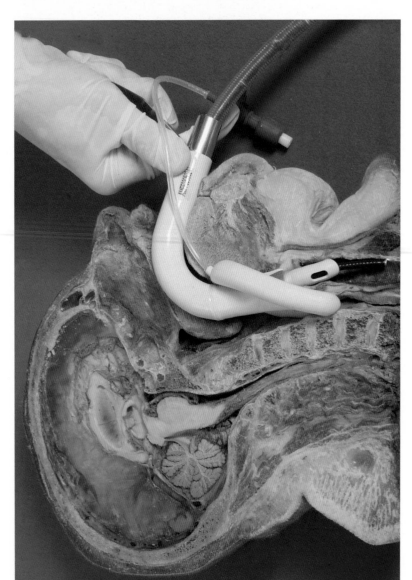

Figure 30.3 ETT advanced over FOB, through ILMA and into glottis.

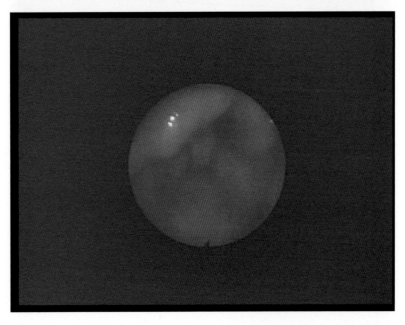

Figure 30.4 Image from FOB: glottic opening.

Figure 30.5 ILMA in place, ventilation confirmed.

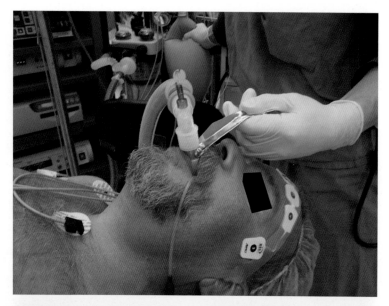

Figure 30.6 ETT is now inserted through the ILMA, up to the 15 cm mark and just beyond, in order to lift the epiglottic elevating bar out of the way of FOB.

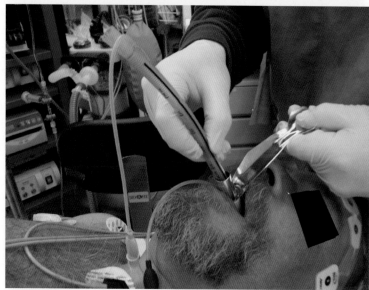

Figure 30.7 FOB is inserted through ETT, into airway, and ETT is advanced over the scope, to an appropriate depth.

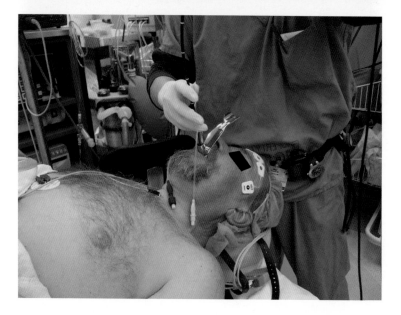

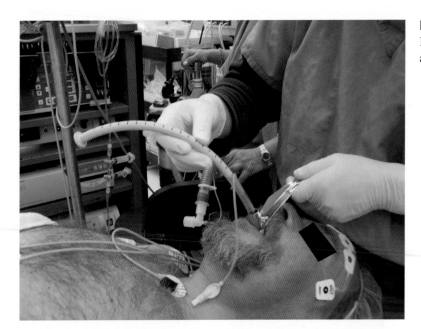

Figure 30.8 The scope is used to confirm ETT position, ventilation is also confirmed, and then the ILMA is removed.

Contraindications: Copious secretions or blood in airway
Inaccessibility of oral cavity
Severe upper airway obstruction

Complications: Complications of both ILMA insertion and FOB intubation are possible with this combination technique (see Chapters 20 and 24)

REFERENCES:

1. Joo HS, Kapoor S, Rose DK, et al. The intubating laryngeal mask airway after induction of general anesthesia versus awake fiberoptic intubation in patients with difficult airways. *Anesth Analg* 2001;92:1342–1346.
2. Ferson DZ, Rosenblatt WH, Johansen MJ, et al. Use of the Intubating LMA-Fastrach in 254 patients with difficult-to-manage airways. *Anesthesiology* 2001;95:1175–1181.

Flexible Fiberoptic Bronchoscope Intubation and the Esophago-Tracheal Combitube

Concept: Although the esophago-tracheal combitube (ETC) has been shown to be reliable for mechanical ventilation for long periods (1), the device is not suitable for long-term intensive care unit (ICU) care, since it neither permits suctioning of the airway nor does it strictly prevent tracheal aspiration of gastric contents. Furthermore, prolonged inflation of the large oropharyngeal balloon could potentially lead to nerve compression in the oral cavity. A patient with difficult ventilation or intubation in whom an ETC is required will likely require definitive tracheal intubation for continued care in the operating room or critical care units. A fiberoptic bronchoscope (FOB) is a viable option for ensuring safe transition from supraglottic to intratracheal ventilation, without removing the lifesaving ETC device until the endotracheal tube (ETT) is securely in place. The ETC is moved to the left side of the mouth, the oropharyngeal balloon is deflated, and the FOB is inserted. After locating the glottis, the larynx and trachea are entered, and the ETT advanced. If desaturation occurs during the procedure, the oropharyngeal balloon can be quickly reinflated, and ventilation initiated, until oxygen saturations once again permit a brief period of apnea.

Evidence: Evidence for this combination of technique is limited to anecdotal reports (2).

Preparations:

Insert ETC (see Chapter 22)
Prepare for FOB (see Chapter 20)
Lubricate ETT, load it onto scope
Anesthetized or unconscious, pre-oxygenated patient in neutral position, with ongoing ventilation via the ETC

Procedure (Figs. 31.1 to 31.3):

Deflate oropharyngeal ETC cuff
Move the ETC to the left side of the mouth
Insert FOB into oral cavity, then pharynx
Visualize the glottis, anterior to the ETC
Advance FOB into glottis, then into trachea
Slide ETT over FOB into trachea
If the ETT cannot be advanced, or the glottis cannot be visualized, the oropharyngeal balloon can be reinflated and ventilation temporarily resumed
Confirm ETT with breath sounds, ETCO$_2$, and chest rise
Secure ETT
Carefully remove the ETC after both cuffs are deflated

Practicality: Because of use of FOB, and crowding in the pharynx from the presence of both devices, this is neither simple nor familiar and requires training and practice
FOB requires logistic support (see Chapter 20)
Not easily portable

Indications: Need for ETT after ETC is utilized for emergent ventilation
Inability to perform direct laryngoscopy for ETT insertion with ETC in place

Contraindications: Copious blood or secretions in airway
Laryngeal trauma

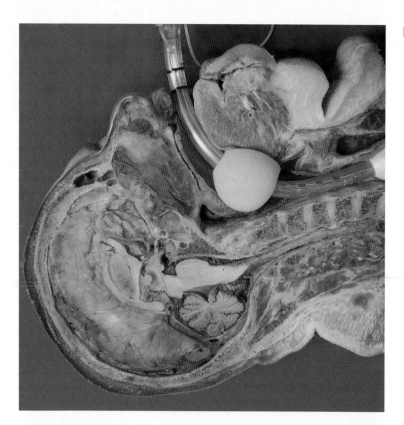

Figure 31.1 ETC in place in cadaver specimen.

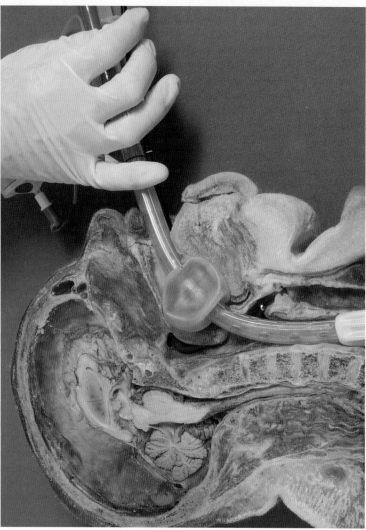

Figure 31.2 Insertion of FOB into pharynx, with oropharyngeal cuff down.

Figure 31.3 FOB inserted into larynx, with ETC in place in simulation laboratory.

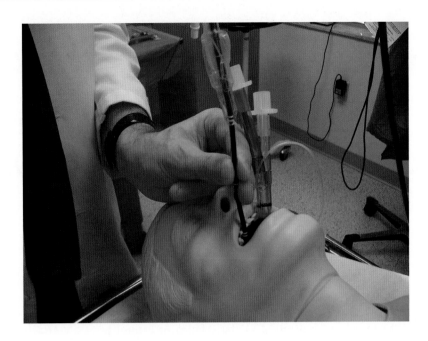

REFERENCES:

1. Frass M. Mechanical ventilation with the esophageal tracheal combitube in the intensive care unit. *Arch Emerg Med* 1987;4:219–223.
2. Ovassapian A. Fiberoptic intubation with Combitube in place. *Anesth Analg* 1993;S315.

Transtracheal Jet Ventilation and Flexible Fiberoptic Bronchoscope Intubation

Concept: Transtracheal Jet Ventilation (TTJV) is rarely used, but remains an important option in the cannot-intubate, cannot-ventilate patient, especially if supraglottic ventilation devices [laryngeal mask airway (LMA), esophageal-tracheal combitube (ETC), perilaryngeal airway (PLA), or laryngeal tube(LT)] have failed or cannot be inserted. After oxygenation and ventilation with TTJV are established, the airway nonetheless remains unprotected. If the patient cannot rapidly be awakened to resume spontaneous ventilation, or if this is contraindicated, an endotracheal tube (ETT) should be placed to guarantee patency of the airway and protect the patient from aspiration of pharyngeal or gastric contents.

Evidence: The combination of these two techniques is supported by anecdotal evidence (1,2). The pressures generated by TTJV may serve to splint open the airway, facilitating fiberoptic bronchoscopy (FOB), while permitting ongoing ventilation during the procedure (1).

Preparation:

Preparation for TTJV (see Chapter 26)
Preparation for FOB (see Chapter 20)
Anesthetized, pre-oxygenated patient in neutral position, with head extension

Procedure (Figs. 32.1 to 32.4):

Place catheter through cricothyroid membrane (CTM) and establish ventilation with TTJV (see Chapter 26)
Remove oral airway, if in place (nasal airways should remain to promote effective exhalation of air)
Attempt direct laryngoscopy (place ETT if glottis visible)
Assistant should continue direct laryngoscopy, to maintain patency of airway for expired gases, or an oral airway (such as Ovassapian airway) can be utilized to facilitate FOB
Additionally, a jaw thrust should be maintained by assistant (in absence of direct laryngoscopy)

Insert FOB into pharynx
Locate glottis, advance FOB into trachea
Avoid hitting or kinking the TTJV catheter
Advance ETT into airway
Remove FOB, confirm that ETT is in trachea
Attach circuit, confirm ETCO$_2$, chest rise, breath sounds
Inflate ETT cuff
Discontinue TTJV, ventilate through ETT
Remove TTJV catheter, fix ETT in place
Note: this procedure can also be applied with nasal FOB, if the mouth cannot be opened

Practicality: Not familiar or simple: requires training and practice assembling components and experience with FOB in patients or simulators
Expensive due to incorporation of FOB
Portability and logistics are an issue due to FOB (see Chapter 20)

Indications: Patient with ongoing TTJV, who requires definitive airway
Patient undergoing TTJV, who has proven to have poor view at direct laryngoscopy
Predicted difficult airway

Contraindications: Copious blood/secretions in airway
Inaccessibility of oral cavity (nasal route may be chosen)
Other contraindications of TTJV (see Chapter 26)

Complications: Complications of both TTJV and FOB intubation are possible with this combined technique (see Chapters 20 and 26)

Figure 32.1 Ongoing TTJV simulated in a cadaver specimen.

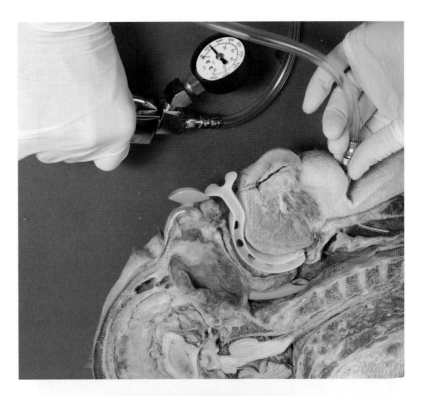

Figure 32.2 Insertion of FOB into larynx, taking care to avoid kinking the TTJV catheter.

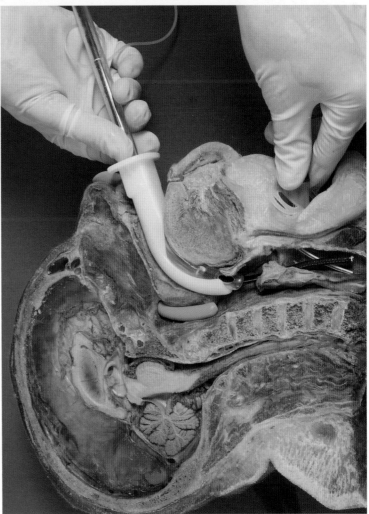

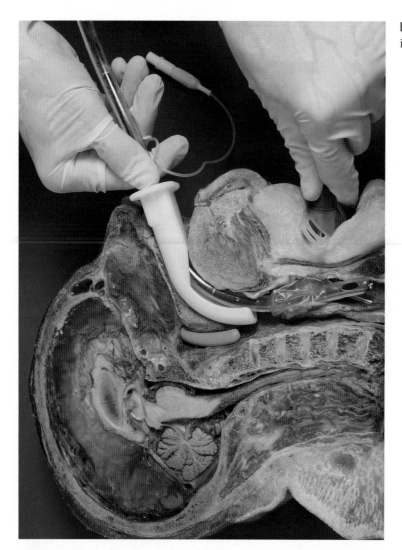

Figure 32.3 Advancement of ETT over FOB, into trachea.

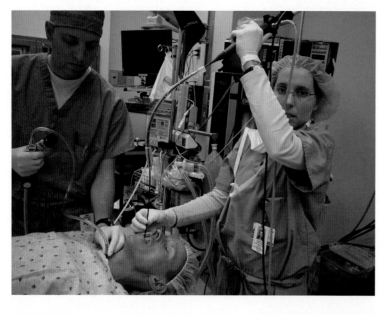

Figure 32.4 In this simulation, ongoing TTJV is shown (note oral and nasal airway in place to allow escape of gas), as a fiberoptic bronchoscope is utilized to carry out oral ETT placement.

REFERENCES:

1. Benumof JL, Scheller MS. The importance of transtracheal jet ventilation in the management of the difficult airway. *Anesthesiology* 1989;71:769–778.

2. Baraka A. Transtracheal jet ventilation during fiberoptic ventilation under general anesthesia. *Anesth Analg* 1986;65:1091–1092.

Cricothyrotomy

Concept: The time-honored means of establishing a rapid, definitive airway when both intubation and ventilation fail is the insertion of a tracheal tube through an incision in the cricothyroid membrane (CTM). Although discouraged in the early part of the 20th century because of complications, chiefly subglottic stenosis, cricothyrotomy was re-established as a safe technique for airway management after publication of the work by Brantigan and Grow, documenting a much lower complication rate than previously believed, among a series of 655 cases (1). The classic technique involves a vertical midline incision over the thyroid and cricoid cartilages, followed by a transverse incision through the cricothyroid membrane. Cricothyrotomy may also be carried out with a single transverse incision through skin and cricothyroid membrane, if the interval is readily palpable (1,2). Because of the small size of the cricothyroid membrane, cricothyrotomy is not indicated in children under the age of eight.

Evidence: Cricothyrotomy is effective for establishing an emergency airway (1), but does carry a risk of acute and chronic complications. Bleeding, failure to secure the airway, and pneumothorax may complicate this procedure, which is typically carried out rapidly and often under duress. Significant rates of long-term complications also occur (3). Reported complication rates for emergent cricothyrotomy are between 10% and 40%. Success rates are quite high in skilled hands, usually above 90%, though these may be considerably lower when carried out by inexperienced personnel (3–5). Because of its invasive and emergent nature, cricothyrotomy is not subject to randomization in trials of airway management, and most evidence is in the form of case series. Recent data suggest that, even in the emergency department, where major trauma and other emergent indications for surgical airways are likely to be higher than in other settings, the incidence of surgical airways approximates only 1% of all intubations (6–8). This is likely due to the success of rapid sequence intubation with direct laryngoscopy as the preferred means of managing the airway (8), the improved training of emergency medicine residents in airway management, and the lower frequency of resuscitation of blunt trauma victims with no detectable vital signs (9). In the face of

falling rates of cricothyrotomy, it has become difficult to maintain proficiency in, and to teach, this essential skill (10).

In the prehospital realm, Spaite described attempted cricothyrotomy in 16 patients with an 88% success rate, as well as a complication rate of 31% (11). Boyle, in a retrospective study of cricothyrotomy by flight nurses in a teaching hospital helicopter transport program, described 69 cricothyrotomy attempts among 2,108 patients transported. The success rate was 98.5%, with a much lower acute complication rate of 8.7% (12).

Preparation (Figs. 33.1 and 33.2):

Prepare tools: 11 blade, small ETT (5.5 or 6.0 cuffed) and hemostat, at a minimum, or a full-fledged tracheostomy set, with tracheostomy tube, if available. A tracheal hook is also desirable.

Test cuff and pilot balloon of ETT or tracheostomy tube, if used. The obturator of the tracheostomy tube should be in place to facilitate insertion.

Locate and palpate CTM

Apply antiseptic solution to anterior neck

Sterile draping (if time allows)

Anesthetized, pre-oxygenated patient in neutral position

Subcutaneous local anesthetic if necessary (if patient is not unconscious)

Procedure (Figs. 33.3 to 33.13):

Grasp thyroid cartilage firmly with long finger and thumb, palpating CTM with index finger of same hand

With the other hand, incise through the skin, vertically, 2 cm to 3 cm, from thyroid prominence to inferior border of cricoid cartilage

Manually retract skin and subcutaneous tissue

Re-identify the CTM with index finger

Incise horizontally, 1 cm to 1.5 cm through lower portion of the CTM

Alternatively, make a single 1.5 cm incision transversely through the skin, subcutaneous tissue, and inferior portion of the CTM, without a vertical incision

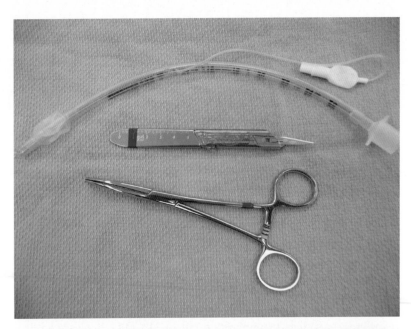

Figure 33.1 "Poor Man's Cricothyromy set": a scalpel, hemostat, and small endotracheal tube can be used to carry out a surgical airway if a formal set is not available.

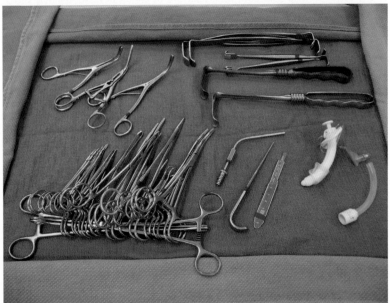

Figure 33.2 Standard Tracheostomy set.

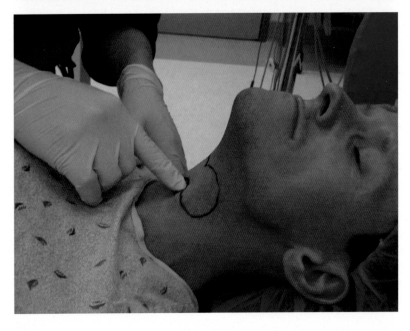

Figure 33.3 Grasping the larynx while palpating the CTM.

Figure 33.4 Dissection of cadaver specimen, revealing the strap muscles covering the larynx and CTM.

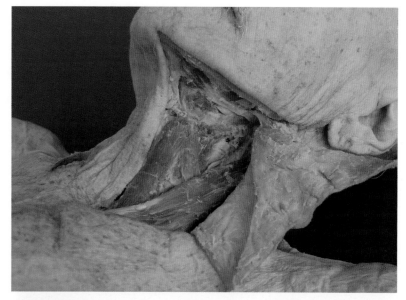

Figure 33.5 Palpation of CTM.

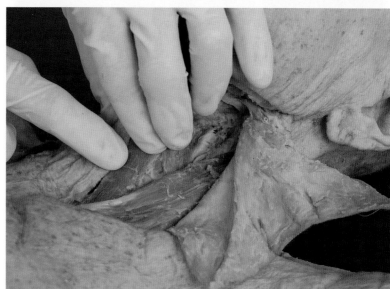

Figure 33.6 Horizontal incision in lower portion of CTM. Vessels crossing the membrane are more likely to be encountered at its cephalad extent.

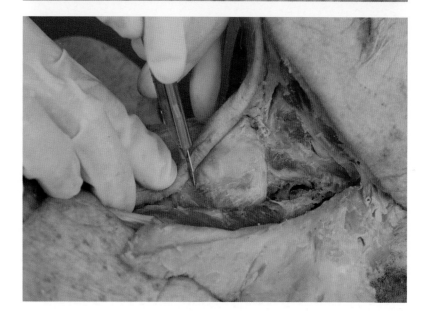

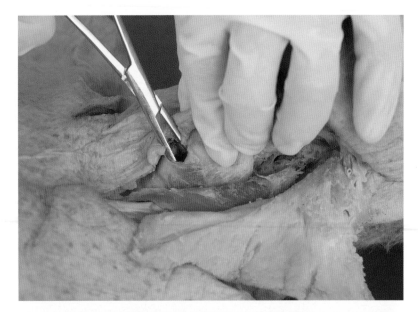

Figure 33.7 Dilator or hemostat is used to enlarge the incision in the CTM after incision (a tracheal hook is helpful to pull the thyroid cartilage upward and towards the patient's head, enhancing the cricothyrotomy before the dilator is placed).

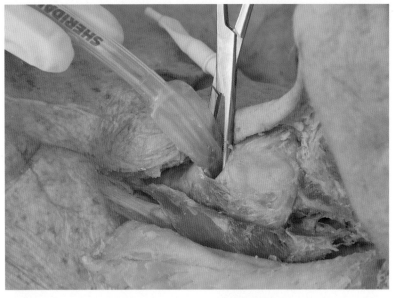

Figure 33.8 Tracheal tube (ETT or tracheostomy tube) is inserted into cricothyroid interval.

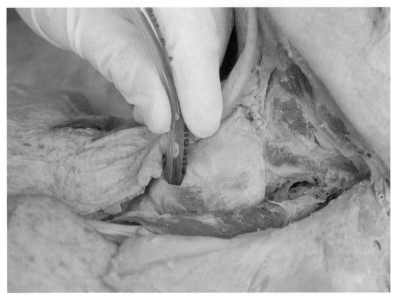

Figure 33.9 After confirmation of ETT (or tracheostomy tube) position in the airway, ventilation can begin.

Figure 33.10 Instead of a single horizontal incision over the CTM, a midline vertical incision can be carried out first, over the thyroid and cricoid cartilages, as shown. (Courtesy of Dr. Samuel Tisherman, Department of Surgery, University of Pittsburgh School of Medicine.)

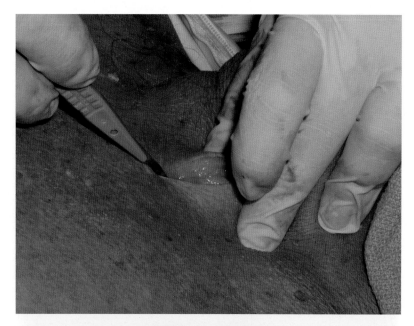

Figure 33.11 After the vertical incision, the skin and subcutaneous tissues are retracted, and the CTM relocated with the index finger. A horizontal incision is then made through the CTM. (Courtesy of Dr. Samuel Tisherman, Department of Surgery, University of Pittsburgh School of Medicine.)

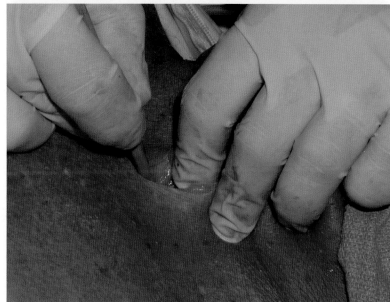

Figure 33.12 A Trousseau dilator (or hemostat) is then utilized to further open the incision through the CTM. (Courtesy of Dr. Samuel Tisherman, Department of Surgery, University of Pittsburgh School of Medicine.)

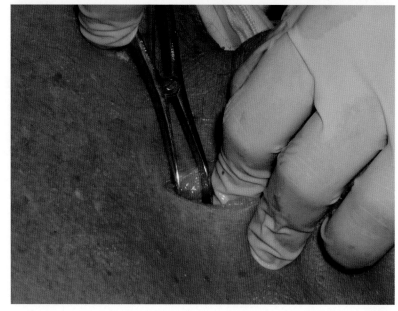

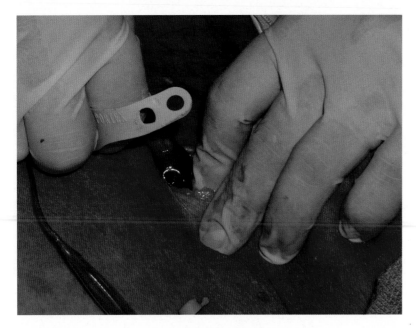

Figure 33.13 As shown, a tracheostomy tube, or an ETT, is inserted into the opening. (Courtesy of Dr. Samuel Tisherman, Department of Surgery, University of Pittsburgh School of Medicine.)

Spread CTM with hemostat, or place a tracheal hook and pull upward on the thyroid cartilage, allowing placement of Trousseau dilator

Dilate the cricothyrotomy opening, from superior to inferior, with hemostat or dilator

Insert ETT or tracheostomy tube between blades of dilator or hemostat. Gentle rotation of dilator as tube is placed facilitates tube entry and advancement in a caudad direction into the trachea.

Remove obturator of tracheostomy tube, inflate cuff of tracheostomy or endotracheal tube, ventilate, and confirm position in airway

Secure tube in place with tape, sutures, or collar and ties

Obtain chest x-ray (CXR) for tube placement

Practicality: Due to declining rates of surgical airways, cricothyrotomy is unfamiliar to most: requires anatomic knowledge and surgical skills; practice with animals or cadavers is desirable
Inexpensive
Portable
"Final common pathway" for life-saving ventilation when all else fails

Indications: Facial, head or neck trauma, when other means of intubation are precluded or impractical
Failure to intubate or ventilate by other methods
Inaccessibility of oral cavity (if nasal intubation fails or is impractical)
Severe upper airway obstruction

Contraindications: Unrecognizable anatomic landmarks

Coagulopathy (relative)
Laryngeal fracture/trauma
Child less than 8 years of age (formal tracheostomy is preferred)
Laryngeal pathology (stenosis, cancer, infection)
Lack of familiarity with technique (relative)

Complications: Bleeding
Infection
ETT misplacement
Laryngeal trauma
Esophageal perforation
Subcutaneous emphysema
Pneumothorax
Voice change, vocal cord injury
Subglottic stenosis
Tracheo-esophageal fistula

REFERENCES:

1. Brantigan CO, Grow JB. Cricothyrotomy: elective use in respiratory problems requiring tracheostomy. *J Thorac and Cardiovasc Surg* 1976;71:72–80.
2. Brantigan CO, Grow JB. Cricothyrotomy revisited again. *Ear Nose Throat J* 1980;59:289–295.
3. Isaacs JH. Emergency cricothyrotomy: long-term results. *Am Surg* 2001;67:346–349.
4. Bair AE, Filbin MR, Kulkarni RG, et al. Failed intubation in the emergency department: analysis of prevalence, rescue techniques and personnel. *J Emerg Med* 2002;23:131–140.
5. Bair AE, Panacek EA, Wisner DH, et al. Cricothyrotomy: a five-year experience at one institution. *J Emerg Med* 2003;24:151–156.
6. Sakles JC, Laurin EG, Rantapaa AA, et al. Airway management

in the emergency department: a one-year study of 610 tracheal intubations. *Ann Emerg Med* 1998;31:325–332.

7. Tayal VS, Riggs RW, Marx JA, et al. Rapid-sequence intubation at an emergency medicine residency: success rate and adverse events during a two-year period. *Acad Emerg Med* 1999;6:31–37.

8. Walls RM, Gurr DE, Kulkarni RG, et al. 6294 Emergency department intubations: second report of the Ongoing National Emergency Airway Registry (NEAR) II study. *Ann Emerg Med* 2000;36:S51.

9. Vissers RJ, Bair AE. Surgical airway techniques, In: Walls RM, ed. *Manual of emergency airway techniques,* 2nd ed. Philadelphia: Lippincott, Williams & Wilkins; 2004:158–182.

10. Chang RS, Hamilton RJ, Carter WA. Declining rate of cricothyrotomy in trauma patients with an emergency medicine residency: implications for skills training. *Acad Emerg Med* 1998;5:247–251.

11. Spaite DW, Maralee J. Prehospital cricothyrotomy: an investigation of indications, technique, complications, and patient outcome. *Ann Emerg Med* 1990;19:279–285.

12. Boyle MF, Hatton D, Sheets C. Surgical cricothyrotomy performed by air ambulance flight nurses: a five year experience. *J Emerg Med* 1993;11:41–45.

Wire-Guided Cricothyrotomy

Concept: Cricothyrotomy may be accomplished with a wire-guided technique, similar to the Seldinger technique for cannulation of vessels. This requires less in the way of surgical skill and experience than does open cricothyrotomy, with a potential for less complications (1.) After puncture of the cricothyroid membrane (CTM) with a thin-walled needle and aspiration of air to confirm intralaryngeal position, a wire is advanced into the airway through the needle, which is then removed (2). After a small incision through the skin, followed by insertion over the wire of an airway catheter and dilator, the dilator is removed, leaving the airway in the trachea. Alternatively, a small incision in the CTM may precede needle placement, to facilitate wire and tracheal tube insertion. The Seldinger technique reduces bleeding and may improve the accuracy of tracheal tube placement (1). Examples of available kits include the Melker Emergency Cricothyrotomy Kit, and Arndt Emergency Cricothyrotomy Set (Cooke Critical Care, Bloomington, IN). There are other commercially available emergency cricothyrotomy sets that do not utilize a guidewire, but rather the dilator/airway is inserted directly over the needle that is used to gain access to the airway. An example is the Patil Emergency Cricothyrotomy Catheter set (Cooke Critical Care, Bloomington, IN).

Evidence: In a randomized, cross-over trial performed on cadavers, Chan compared the open technique of cricothyrotomy to the Melker wire-guided method (3). Of the participating physicians, 94% preferred the wire-guided technique, while the overall success rate was similar for both methods. Eisenberger reported that inexperienced clinicians attempting to perform cricothyrotomy on cadavers had a success rate in the range of only 60% to 70% with either technique (4).

Preparation (Fig. 34.1):

Same as for cricothyrotomy (see Chapter 33)
Open kit, test-fit components (syringe, needle, wire, tracheostomy tube, and obturator/dilator)
Palpate and mark CTM
Anesthetized, or unconscious, pre-oxygenated patient (also, the technique may be carried out in a conscious patient, with local anesthesia injected into the skin and subcutaneous tissue over the cricothyroid membrane)

Procedure (for Melker Emergency Cricothyrotomy Kit) (Figs. 34.2 to 34.6):

Grasp larynx firmly, holding it immobile with thumb and long finger; identify the CTM with the tip of the index finger
Puncture CTM with thin-walled needle attached to a syringe containing saline or water, aiming 45 degrees to caudad
Aspirate air bubbles to confirm needle in airway
Thread wire through needle
Remove needle
Use scalpel to enlarge opening around wire (some authors recommend preceding needle cannulation of CTM with a 1 cm, vertical incision, to facilitate dilator passage)
Pass dilator/airway over wire into airway
Remove dilator, inflate cuff of tracheostomy tube
Attach breathing circuit to cricothyrotomy tube, begin ventilation
Confirm with $ETCO_2$, breath sounds, chest rise
Tie or suture the tube in place

Practicality: Inexpensive
Portable
Unfamiliar and complex: requires training and practice
"Final common pathway" for life-saving ventilation when all else fails

Indications: Facial, head, or neck trauma, where other means of intubation are precluded or impractical
Inaccessibility of oral cavity (if nasal route is not practical)
Failure to intubate or ventilate by other methods
Severe upper airway obstruction

Figure 34.1 Components of Melker cricothyrotomy kit.

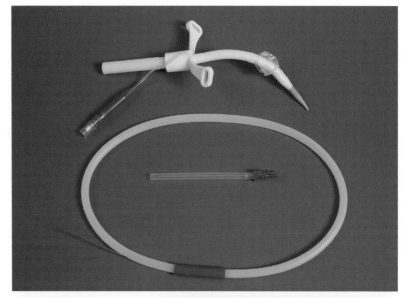

Figure 34.2 Needle puncture through the CTM.

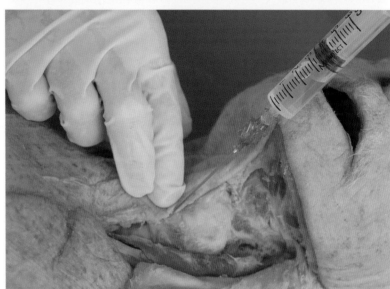

Figure 34.3 After the wire is introduced, the tracheal tube and dilator are threaded over the wire.

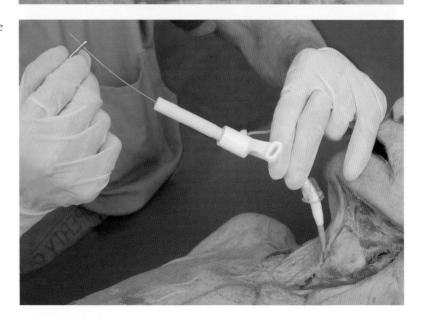

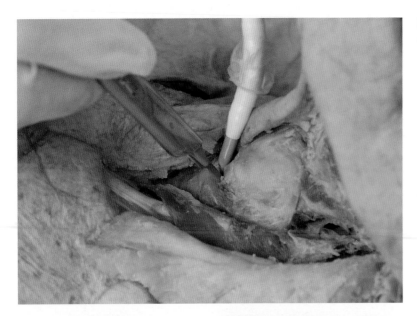

Figure 34.4 The opening in the CTM is enlarged with a scalpel.

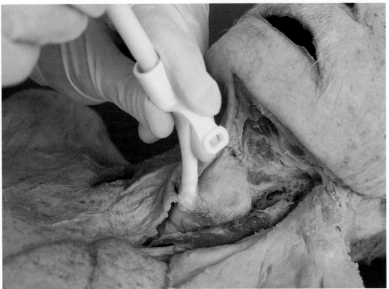

Figure 34.5 The airway and dilator are advanced into the airway.

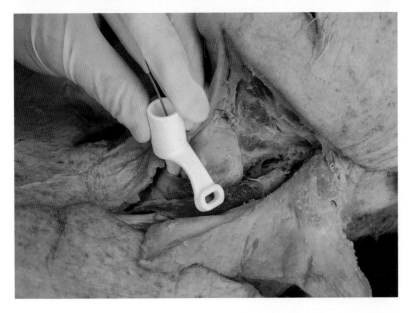

Figure 34.6 The dilator is now removed with the wire, and ventilation can begin after position of the tracheal tube in the airway is confirmed.

Contraindications: Unrecognizable anatomic
landmarks
Child less than 8 years of age
(formal tracheostomy is preferred)
Coagulopathy (relative)
Laryngeal fracture/trauma
Lack of familiarity with the
technique
Laryngeal pathology (stenosis,
cancer, infection)

Complications: Bleeding
Infection
ETT misplacement with failed
ventilation
Laryngeal trauma
Esophageal perforation
Subcutaneous emphysema
Pneumothorax

Subglottic stenosis
Voice change, vocal cord injury
Tracheoesophageal fistula

REFERENCES:

1. Melker RJ, Florete, Jr. OG. Percutaneous dilational cricothyrotomy and tracheostomy. In: Benumof JL, ed. *Airway management, principles and practice.* St. Louis: Mosby; 1996:
484–512.

2. Jackson IJB, Choudhry AK, Ryan DW, et al. Minitracheotomy
Seldinger–assessment of a new technique. *Anesthesia* 1991;
46:475–477.

3. Chan TC, Vilke Gm, Bramwell KJ, et al. Comparison of wire-
guided cricothyrotomy versus standard surgical cricothyrotomy technique. *J Emerg Med* 1999;17:957–962.

4. Eisenberger P, Laczika K, List M, et al. Comparison of
conventional surgical versus Seldinger technique emergency
cricothyrotomy performed by inexperienced clinicians.
Anesthesiology 2000;92:687–690.

Index

Page numbers followed by a t indicate a table while those followed by an f indicate figure.